The Individual Service Funds Handbook

Implementing Personal Budgets in Provider Organisations

HELEN SANDERSON AND ROBIN MILLER

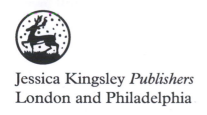

Jessica Kingsley *Publishers*
London and Philadelphia

First published in 2015
by Jessica Kingsley Publishers
73 Collier Street
London N1 9BE, UK
and
400 Market Street, Suite 400
Philadelphia, PA 19106, USA

www.jkp.com

Library of Congress Cataloging in Publication Data
Sanderson, Helen, 1965-
  The individual service funds handbook : implementing personal budgets in
provider organisations / Helen Sanderson and Robin Miller.
    pages cm
 Includes bibliographical references and index.
 ISBN 978-1-84905-423-2 (alk. paper)
 1. Medical savings accounts--Great Britain. 2. Personalized medicine-
-Great Britain. 3. Medical care--Great Britain. I. Title.
 RA416.5.G7S257 2015
 338.4'33621--dc23
                          2014021852

British Library Cataloguing in Publication Data
A CIP catalogue record for this book is available from the British Library

ISBN 9 780 85700 792 6
eISBN 9 780 85700 792 6

Printed and bound in Great Britain

Contents

Section 2 Key Issues and Learning in Implementation

Section 3 ISFs: Moving to the Future

Acknowledgements

We would like to thank the many people who took time out of their busy jobs to share their experiences and contribute their invaluable learning to the completion of this book.

There are a few people who require particular thanks: Professor Roger Ellis from Bucks New University; May Lee and Sean Lindley from Certitude; Sian Hoolahan from Choice Support; Ceri Shepherd from Look Ahead Care and Support; Bob Timmins and Sarah Sims from Real Life Options; Ben Harrison from United Response; Jo Greenbank and Paul Pargeter from Dimensions; Lisa Martin from Bruce Lodge, Borough Care Ltd; Ruth Gorman from Imagine, Act and Succeed (IAS); and Suzie and Jennie Franklin.

We are grateful to Gill Bailey and Michelle Livesley for all their help with the stories and examples, and to Julie Barclay for the diagrams.

The information about the learning from IAS was taken from a paper by Owen Cooper, Helen Sanderson, Ruth Gorman, Michelle Livesley and Terry Keely, titled 'What are we learning about Individual Service Funds?' (2008). This book builds on the paper 'Choice and control for all' by Helen Sanderson, Sam Bennett, Simon Stockton and Jaimee Lewis, published by Groundswell Partnership (2011). The 'Working Together for Change' example is taken from the book *Making Individual Service Funds Work for People with Dementia Living in Care Homes: How It Works in Practice* by Helen Sanderson and Gill Bailey with Lisa Martin, also published by Jessica Kingsley Publishers (2014). All diagrams in this book were developed by Helen Sanderson Associates and are used with permission.

Introduction

Individual Service Funds (ISFs) are an important way to deliver personalisation. Before we explain why we chose to focus this book on ISFs, it is important to explore what we understand by personalisation. There is no one starting point at which we can say that 'personalisation' as an approach on which to base care services was proposed and agreed. It is both a 'top-down' and 'bottom-up' initiative which has been championed at the grassroots level by people receiving support, but which has also been pushed forward by governments.[1] The 'bottom-up' is the leadership by disabled people and their allies that extends back to the United States in the 1970s in which disabled people developed the independent living movement as a vehicle to promote and advocate for their right to have control over their lives. The movement was picked up in the UK by people with physical disabilities living in residential care homes who wanted the opportunity to live in the community and not an institution. There was increasing anger about both the quality of care and the ethical basis of confining people with a learning disability within long-stay hospitals, and challenges to the dominance of medical models within psychiatry. Along with concerned clinicians, practitioners and academics, much of these campaigns were being instigated by newly formed self-advocacy and survivor groups. The Valuing People national strategy for learning disability[2] published in 2001 is often seen as an important landmark in which national policy adopted these principles, with its emphasis on 'rights, independence, choice and inclusion' and promotion of person-centred planning as a process through which people could be enabled to determine their own futures.

Accompanying these grassroots pressures were changes in thinking about the way in which public services were to be delivered. Based partly on political ideology and partly on frustration that the public sector was resistant to change, there was a move towards the role of government being to coordinate and procure support rather than provide services directly. Citizens would be seen as having individual rights, but also responsibilities, to contribute and make wise decisions about their own lifestyles and families. Rather than public services being improved through control from the centre, markets would be created in which people receiving support could choose from a range of providers and thus drive quality up and drive price down. This would enable private-sector organisations to deliver more public services and thus bring in new innovations in technology and higher standards of 'customer service'. Third-sector organisations would also take on a greater delivery role through which they could extend voluntary action and embed their strong values and beliefs. In practical terms, these changes in political beliefs led to the externalisation of many local authority and NHS-run care facilities and the introduction of 'care management' as a process through which an individual would have their needs assessed and services procured to meet those needs.

Whilst the 'top-down' and 'bottom-up' forces may have begun from a different set of interests and pressures, there was a 'meeting in the middle' regarding core elements that have become associated with personalisation – the rights of the individual to a responsive service and individuals having the opportunity and expectation to contribute their own assets and resources. Bringing these elements together were a number of key 'policy entrepreneurs' who passionately

---

1   Needham, C. (2011) *Personalising Public Services: Understanding the Personalisation Narrative.* Bristol: Policy Press.
2   Department of Health (2001) *Valuing People: A New Strategy for Learning Disability for the 21st Century.* London: HM Government. Available at www. gov.uk/government/uploads/system/uploads/attachment_data/file/250877/5086.pdf, accessed on 12 June 2014.

believed that the previous care system had lost its way and this was an opportunity to introduce fundamental changes to the basic principles and processes on which it was operating.

Personalisation is therefore more than government policy, and there are those who are concerned that the more radical potential of personalisation may be lost if governments are able to take on primary 'ownership' of the concept. Policy documents are, however, still a useful reflection on what is meant by personalisation within different countries at a set time period. Whilst it is not possible to know from the outside exactly how end definitions were reached, governments who have taken on the concept appear to have sought to engage people who access services and their representative groups within the development process. For instance, in Scotland, the Changing Lives Social Work Review had a user and carer panel who were able to contribute to the discussions about the purpose and future of social work. This panel was able to clearly articulate the hopes of what could be achieved through personalisation, and this informed the objectives of personalisation that were subsequently defined by the Changing Lives Service Development Group (Box I.1).

To achieve whole-scale change in a care system and correct flaws that have been built up over many decades is clearly going to take time and require coordinated and planned actions. The Scottish Association of Directors of Social Work identified a set of principles that would need to be adopted by those responsible for planning, designing and providing care services (Box I.2).

Box I.1 Scottish perspectives on personalisation

The user and carer panel of the Changing Lives Social Work Review states:[3]

> We expect services to make a positive difference to our lives. We are people first. The outcomes we want include having power and control, being able to take risks and contribute to society. This means that there needs to be a shift in power away from people who commission and provide services to service users and carers.

The Scottish Government states:[4]

> [Personalisation enables] the individual alone, or in groups, to find the right solutions for them and to participate in the delivery of a service. From being a recipient of services, citizens can become actively involved in selecting and shaping the services they receive.

These principles are mirrored in the Putting People First initiative in England[5] which identified four areas that have to be addressed if personalisation is to be made a reality:

- *Universal services.* Mainstream services such as health, leisure, education, housing and others should be accessible to everyone, including those with disabilities and different forms of communication. These services enable people to stay independent and healthy, to make the same choices as the rest of the community and to avoid requiring specialist care and support services.

---

3   Scottish Executive (2006) *Changing Lives: Report of the 21st Century Social Work Review*. Edinburgh: The Scottish Government.
4   Service Development Group of Changing Lives (2009) *Personalisation: A Shared Understanding*. Edinburgh: The Scottish Government.
5   Department of Health (2001) *Putting People First: A Shared Vision and Commitment to the Transformation of Adult Social Care*. London: HM Government.

Box I.2 The principles of personalisation

The principles of personalisation are as follows:

- The right to self-determination and citizenship is for everyone.

- The public have the right to expect quality, timely and easily accessible information and advocacy services to support them to exercise choice over the support they receive.

- Social work must play its part with others in creating a system that leads to a better life for all citizens and reduces the need for reliance upon formal services.

- People have the right to make their own decisions about risk, unless there is a statutory reason to prevent it. It should be presumed that individuals have the capacity to make balanced judgements about factors that affect their quality of life.

- Personalisation is not the sole interest or responsibility of any one agency. Corporate ownership is required to lead whole-system change. The full involvement of health services in delivering the agenda is of key importance.

- Social work services cannot effectively contribute to a personalised approach without a knowledgeable, skilled and empowered workforce that is committed to the agenda and the values and principles that underpin it.

(After Association of Directors of Social Work)[6]

- *Early intervention and prevention.* Ideally we want to prevent people from requiring care through helping them to stay well and avoid accidents such as falls. When someone does have an illness or trauma, it is important that they be able to regain their skills and confidence so that they can resume previous interests and responsibilities and maintain their chosen level of independence. Whilst reablement and rehabilitative services have important roles, the encouragement and support of friends or neighbours, starting to exercise and eating well can make a major difference. Similarly, if someone develops a long-term health care condition, they can often take steps to reduce the impact on their quality of life and prevent any further deterioration. This could be through information, training and support from someone else who already lives with the condition.

- *Choice and control.* When people do need care it is vital that it be based around what support they want and when, rather than what suits the services and the staff. This requires good information about what funding they are entitled to, the options for managing it and how they can spend it. It also means that services have to be willing to listen to the person, to keep their focus on responding to their needs and wishes and to enable them to make decisions and take risks.

- *Social capital.* Families and communities are made up of bonds between individuals and groups, and through these bonds we are able to provide practical support, give each other comfort and enjoy interests and passions. They also enable us to have a say over what will happen in our communities and areas. Many people who access care are excluded from

---

6   Association of Directors of Social Work (2009) *Personalisation: Principles, Challenges and a New Approach.* Available at www.adsw.org.uk/home.aspx?MicrositeID=1&LevelxID=39, accessed on 12 June 2014.

these bonds, and this means that they can miss out on these opportunities. It also means that the community is not able to benefit from their contributions

Money and personalisation

Personalisation is about much more than money; however, enabling people to be clear about what public funding is available to them and giving them the opportunity to have greater control over how this funding is spent is an important part of achieving personalisation in practice. In part this is due to the perceived 'power' of money, in that deciding what to buy and who will provide it may give the person concerned greater influence over a provider than if they receive funding from a third party. It is also tied in with the notion of being 'citizens' who are entitled to receive support due to our contribution to, and membership in, a collective society, rather than it being available because 'professionals' have decided that it would be to our benefit (often called the 'professional gift' model). Social care has taken a lead, with all people who are eligible for publicly funded adult social care services being informed about the budget that they are entitled to receive. Following a national pilot programme, personal budgets are also now to be available in England in relation to NHS-funded health care services.

With both health and social care budgets there are three principal mechanisms connected with this funding: direct payments, commissioner managed and third-party managed (Box I.3).

Box I.3 Financial processes in personalisation

The financial processes in personalisation are as follows:

- *Commissioner managed.* The public body retains the cash to which the individual is entitled and purchases services on their behalf. The expectation is that the individual makes decisions about what services they will receive and who will provide these services.

- *Direct payment.* The cash to which the individual is entitled is transferred from the public body to the individual's bank account. This cash can be used to purchase services or in other ways that would meet the individual's assessed needs and achieve the outcomes agreed with the public body.

- *Third-party managed.* If the individual is not able to personally manage their budget, the cash can be transferred to a third party to be managed on their behalf.

The main focus for these new financial options are people who are living in the community and not in congregate settings. This excludes (or perhaps, more accurately, neglects) those who are living in residential care homes and/or access services that receive funding to provide support to a set number of people (commonly day services or supported-living schemes). For these individuals, the potential power that arises from being more in control of their allocated funding has therefore been denied. Individual Service Funds are a means of transferring this power, and the life-enhancing opportunities that it can enable to such individuals. In relation to the financial processes outlined above, ISFs can be seen as third-party managed budgets held by the main provider of the support to an individual.

For a provider to hold a budget and ensure that its use is being tailored to the wishes of the individual receiving support presents a number of complex and potentially difficult issues. Can organisations separate out the funding to which an individual is eligible if the service is purchased and provided on a block basis? Will the provider be able to change the working practices and patterns of staff to respond to how the person wants to live and be supported? Will the organisation and its staff be content for the individual to take part or all of their funding elsewhere if they are not fully satisfied with the service that they receive? How can this be done at scale across a number of different services?

This book seeks to explore these issues through reflecting on the experiences of organisations that have made progress in introducing ISFs in the UK, and that are working towards implementing these ISFs at scale. In Section 1 we explore in more detail what is meant by ISFs and how they can be authentically developed through introducing robust and person-centred processes that ensure that the person concerned is the focus of the funding, planning and delivery of the service. In Section 2 we consider how these individual processes can be introduced in an organisation and made relevant to people with different needs and in service contexts. This includes people using mental health services, people living with dementia in a care home and people with learning disabilities living in group homes. In Section 2 we also learn about the potential for assistive technology to support the process and how the impact of ISFs can be measured. In Section 3 we look to the future and examples of how ISFs have been introduced within a wider range of services, and conclude the section, and the book, with the key points of learning regarding the implementation of ISFs.

Throughout this book we draw on the experience and perspectives of six organisations, outlining what led them to consider ISFs within their services. These accounts are based on the perspectives of the organisations themselves and are therefore presented as a series of individual stories. We use the term 'the organisations' to refer to these organisations as a collective group.

The organisations' stories

BOROUGH CARE LTD

Borough Care Ltd is an industrial and provident society with charitable status based in Stockport. Established in 1993, it now has 11 residential care services which provide long-term care, short break and day care. It supports older people, including those with dementia or a high level of care needs.

The commissioner of services for older people in Stockport was aware that personalisation had largely been considered in relation to people who were living in the community and this meant that people living in care homes may not have been able to benefit. They were also keen to understand how the principles could be applied for people who were living with dementia, and they decided to look for a local provider who would be willing to work with them to explore this in practice. They sent a copy of a book describing how these principles had been applied in residential care[7] to all providers of services for people living with dementia in Stockport and asked for expressions of interest in being part of a pilot project.

There was one expression of interest – Borough Care Ltd. The commissioner organised a half-day meeting with Helen Sanderson Associates, key staff from Stockport Council and Borough Care Ltd to talk about the potential project. The deputy CEO and six home managers attended, together with the contacts and quality officer, workforce development officer and commissioner from Stockport Council. From this meeting, Borough Care Ltd decided to focus the project

---

7   Scown, S. and Sanderson, H. (2011) *Making It Personal for Everyone*. Stockport: HSA Press.

on Bruce Lodge. The project was to use the principles of ISFs with the 43 people living with dementia at Bruce Lodge.

CERTITUDE

Certitude has worked across London since 1990 and provides personalised support for over 1000 people with learning disabilities, autism and mental health needs, and their family carers. As a charity incorporated as an industrial and provident society, Certitude delivers a wide range of community- and accommodation-based services.

Prior to considering ISFs, Certitude had already undertaken considerable work in relation to person-centred working in their learning disability services, and recovery approaches within their mental health services. Keen to develop more personalised services, Certitude decided that it needed to do more to make the support planning process and the resources available to individuals more transparent. In relation to the broader policy environment, Certitude determined that not all individuals (such as those within shared services, e.g. residential care) would be able to access personal budgets and that others who would be eligible for a personal budget would not be able to manage it due to a lack of capacity or a lack of non-paid relationships.

Certitude was looking, therefore, for means to further personalise their services and ensure that all individuals who access services can benefit from the opportunity to manage and direct their care and support budgets. Due to the considerable pressures on local authority and health commissioners, Certitude was also keen to be able to achieve these changes without having to rely too heavily on their purchasers, as it was recognised that their capacity might be limited. Certitude decided to initially trial ISFs in eight services across three local authority boroughs. These were six care homes and supported-living projects for people with a learning disability that were funded through block contracts, and two care homes for people with mental health issues. As the plan was for ISFs to be made available within all services, these initial projects were seen as 'prototypes' rather than 'pilots'.

CHOICE SUPPORT

Choice Support is a social care charity that was first envisaged in 1984 when a consortium was developed across statutory, voluntary and housing sectors to facilitate the closure of a long-stay hospital for people with a learning disability. It now works throughout much of England, supporting disabled and disadvantaged people, including those with learning disabilities, mental health needs, physical disabilities and homeless people. Its initial interest in relation to ISFs was centred on a block contract for people with a learning disability. This had been in place for over 20 years in relation to services costing nearly £7 million.

When the ISF project began, these services were being used by 83 people. Having a block contract had advantages for Choice Support, in that they could move staff around to address pressures in particular services, had a guaranteed level of income and involved relatively straightforward invoicing arrangements; however, the organisation was concerned that the block arrangement meant that the aspirations of the people concerned were not considered in the allocation of funding, that changes in their life and needs were not being reviewed and that the funding available to support each person was not transparent. Overall, the block arrangement seemed to be in conflict with their principles of choice and support, as it restricted individuals' ability to shape what support they received and who provided it. Whilst the organisation had already taken steps to become more personalised in their practice, there was a consensus that a plateau had been reached and a new catalyst was needed to enable the staff to make further improvements.

In addition to these issues, there was a requirement by the purchaser that they reduce the costs of the contract by almost 30 per cent. Such levels of savings could not be achieved without Choice Support radically reviewing how it delivered these services. Choice Support also had a good relationship with the purchaser, which gave the organisation confidence that it would be able to work collaboratively with the local authority and could trust the local authority to be supportive.

DIMENSIONS

Dimensions is a not-for-profit organisation that began in 1975. It is the largest organisation that we looked at, supporting over 3000 people with a learning disability or autism across England and Wales. Dimensions offers a range of support services to children and adults of all ages, including those with autism and complex needs, and their carers.

Like many providers, Dimensions supports large numbers of people who live, and will probably continue to live, in what can be described as traditional (shared) services (sometimes called residential care homes or group homes). While some services provide very good support, there is no escaping the fundamental flaws: the people have not chosen who they live with, and they have a limited choice about who supports them and how their time is spent because the team on duty works with everyone. This was therefore a tension with Dimensions' wholehearted support for the 'personalisation' agenda and its emphasis on enabling people to have a greater say over the services they receive and how these services are delivered.

For Dimensions the question therefore was clear: how could the organisation help people in traditional services take control of their funding and determine and control their own support? Dimensions decided that it was necessary to change the way the organisation did things if the people it supported were going to realise more choice and control in their lives, and fundamental to this change was people knowing and controlling their budgets. From the outset Dimensions was clear that whilst having choice and control over money does not guarantee a better life for people using services, it is a fundamental starting point to make this happen.

LOOK AHEAD CARE AND SUPPORT

Look Ahead Care and Support (hereafter referred to as Look Ahead) is a charitable housing association that provides specialist support and care services to people with a variety of needs across London and the South East. One of its services is Coventry Road, an accommodation-based housing support service for people with mental health problems. At the time of the ISF project the service was jointly commissioned by the local authority (through its Supporting People funding) and the primary care trusts. The commissioners and Look Ahead were interested in exploring how the principles of personalisation could be offered to a broader range of people who use services, including those in tenancy support services and those who were block funded. The pilot project sought to develop a cost-effective model in which the continued need to ensure safety and promote recovery were achieved alongside increased personal choice and control for customers.

The trial at Coventry Road ended in 2010, and following reductions in the Supporting People budget, it has been difficult to sustain the 'core and flexi' model that was introduced. The learning has been used, though, in the development of the mental health rehabilitation service. This service has 11 self-contained flats for people with complex mental health problems, including those with severe depression, psychosis and a personality disorder. It is commissioned by the Clinical Commissioning Group, and Look Ahead sub-contracts with an NHS Mental Health Foundation Trust for clinical support. Personal allocations of funding were built into the funding from the outset.

REAL LIFE OPTIONS

Real Life Options is a national voluntary organisation that was started in 1992 in London and supports over 750 people with a learning disability or autism across the UK. It had won two contracts in Birmingham to manage residential care homes that had been set up as part of the closure of long-stay hospitals. Real Life Options recognised that whilst the basic care within the homes was acceptable, there was considerable opportunity to improve the quality of life of the people who were living within them. Birmingham City Council agreed with the need to improve the quality of the homes but also required Real Life Options to achieve financial savings. Real Life Options wanted to demonstrate that it was possible to improve quality and save money in these services through working in partnership with other organisations and the commissioners.

To deliver the Transformation of Residential Care Homes (TORCH) programme, Real Life Options therefore sought to build on previous work in developing person-centred practices, and to partner with telecare provider Tunstall in relation to deploying assistive technology equipment within care homes. Real Life Options also introduced the principles of ISFs as a third element (alongside person-centred practices and assistive technology) to the TORCH programme on the basis that having greater transparency and control over resources would be further lever for change. As well as improving the lives of people living in these homes, Real Life Options wanted to learn as an organisation from their experiences so that they could roll out positive practice within their other services. They also wanted to share learning and good practice with other companies and local authorities. To assist the project team to understand the impacts of the changes and draw out the main learning points, Real Life Options commissioned the University of Birmingham to work with the organisation in evaluating the programme.

In addition to these six organisations, we also draw on examples and learning from Positive Futures in Northern Ireland as well as Imagine, Act and Succeed in Greater Manchester. Positive Futures supports adults, children and families, and is the first provider in Northern Ireland to explore ISFs. Ruth Gorman, Owen Cooper and Michelle Livesley developed some of the very early work around ISFs, and developed useful papers describing their learning.[8]

---

8   Cooper, O., Sanderson, H., Gorman, R., Livesley, M. and Keely, T. (2008) *What are we Learning About Individual Service Funds?* Available at www.supportplanning.org/Support_Planning_Downloads/SP_40_What_are_we_ learning_about_ Individual_Service_Funds_Sept_08.pdf, accessed 12 June 2014.

The Individual Service Fund Process

Chapter 1
Individual Service Funds

Introduction

An Individual Service Fund (ISF) is one way that individuals can have greater choice and control through a personal budget. Rather than the individual, their carer or a public-sector organisation holding the individual's budget, the money is managed by a provider organisation on the individual's behalf. The concept of an ISF was first used in Scotland by Inclusion Glasgow and Partners for Inclusion, supporting people with learning disabilities in the late 1990s.[1] ISFs were part of In Control's model of self-directed support, and from 2005 to 2007,[2] the councils involved in the UK government's individual budget pilot started to look at ISFs to enable people to have greater choice within commissioned or in-house services. Today ISFs are an important way that personal budgets can work in practice within provider organisations. In this chapter we look at the relationship between different funding processes and definitions as well as best practice standards regarding ISFs, and we describe the process of developing an ISF from allocation through to person-centred review.

Funding mechanisms and ISFs

Broadly, there are three mechanisms through which an ISF can be organised (see Figure 1.1, page 20) and which can be applied to all or part of the funding to which someone is entitled from the public sector or from their own resources. The first mechanism is that the individual in receipt of a direct payment transfers all or part of this cash to the organisation that provides care and support to the individual. The second mechanism is that the public body providing the funding sets up a contract with a provider to manage part or all of the budget to which the individuals accessing the service are entitled. The third mechanism is that an individual who is funding their care from their own resources and who does not receive financial assistance from the public sector transfers cash to the provider to manage on their behalf. (We discuss these mechanisms in more detail later in the chapter.)

Whichever form the ISF takes, there are a number of key elements that must be in place (Box 1.1, page 18).

---

1 Poll, C., Duffy, S., Hatton, C., Sanderson, H. and Routledge, M. (2006) *A Report on In Control's First Phase 2003–2005*. London: In Control Publications.
2 Poll *et al.* (2006).

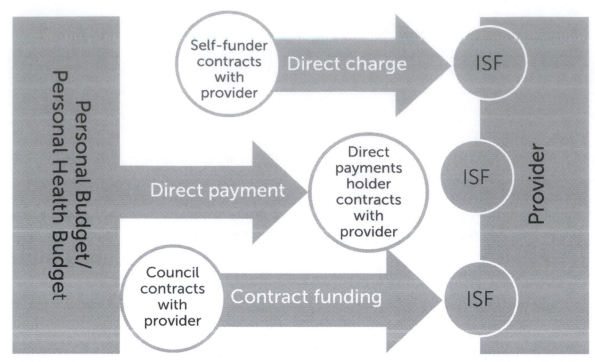

Figure 1.1 The relationship between the different funding mechanisms (based on Bennett and Miller 2009)[3]

Box 1.1 Key features of ISFs

The key features of ISFs are as follows:

- All or part of a personal budget is held by a provider on an individual's behalf, and the money is restricted for use on that person's support and accounted for accordingly.

- No specific tasks are predetermined so that the personal budget holder is empowered to plan with the provider the who, how, where, when and what of any support provided.

- There is flexibility to roll money or support over into future weeks or months and to bank support for particular purposes.

- The ISF is accompanied by written information that clearly explains the arrangement and confirms any management costs to come from the personal budget.

- There is portability, so the personal budget holder can choose to use the money in a different way or with a different provider.

(From Bennett and Miller)[4]

---

3   Bennett, S. and Miller, C. (2009) *Contracting for Personalised Outcomes: Learning from Emerging Practice.* London: UK Department of Health.
4   Bennett and Miller (2009).

As you can see from these key features, it is vital that there is clarity about the budget that is held on the person's behalf by the provider, transparency about how this money is used and clarity regarding any management costs that will be incurred. The person should be central to identifying what outcomes they want to achieve from this funding and to the decision-making process over how these outcomes are achieved in practice. There must be flexibility in the way that the budget is used so that the person can choose to spend it on a regular basis or save it in order to buy or access something more expensive. The individual should be able to continue to use the main provider to deliver any connected support or to choose to employ an alternative provider to deliver part of this support. They must also be able to spend the money in a different way. This could be in relation to using community resources to pursue a particular hobby or leisure interest or to undertake learning in order to develop a new skill or talent. The provider must be accountable to the person for this budget and keep them informed about what is available and what has been spent and on what.

Figure 1.2 shows another way to describe the features of ISFs. This model draws on our understanding of how truly personalised support can work for people, is grounded in the language used by the disability movement to describe what should be different in services and was produced together with people with support needs as well as their carers and families. It consists of a number of first-person statements for what people might be saying if each element were working well.[5]

Individual Service Funds

WHAT "I can use my hours/budget flexibly and can choose what I am supported with."

WHERE "I am supported where it makes sense for me, at home and out and about."

WHO "I choose who I want to support me, my support worker knows me and I know them."

WHEN "I get support on the days and at the times that are right for me."

HOW "I choose how I am supported and my support workers know this is important to me."

CO-PRODUCTION "I am fully involved in decisions about my own support and how the wider service develops."

Figure 1.2 Good practice in Individual Service Funds (from Sanderson et al.)[6]

5   Sanderson, H., Bennett, S., Stockton, S. and Lewis, J. (2012) *Choice and Control for All: The Role of Individual Service Funds in Delivering Fully Personalised Care and Support (p.8).* London: Groundswell Partnership.
6   Sanderson *et al.* (2012).

Starting points for ISFs

Now let's go back to the current funding arrangements in the UK and look at the three ways that an organisation can develop ISFs in greater detail. The first way is that they arise through 'micro-commissioning' in which the commissioner, the person or their family ask the provider to manage all or part of their personal budget on their behalf. In this scenario a new service is being developed to respond to what is important to the individuals, their outcomes and aspirations within the allocated budget. It requires the person concerned and their circle of support to be involved in decisions about how best to spend the budget and what is, and is not, achievable within the resources available. This also relates to people who are self-funding their care. (In Chapter 13 we describe an example of a circle commissioning their service from a provider using an ISF.)

The second approach is where a provider receives individual funding for the individuals who access their service through separate contracts with the commissioner(s), but this funding is pooled to run the service as a whole. Even if people have some elements of individual support funded by the commissioner, they have little control over what outcomes this funding should achieve or how it is spent in practice. Similar to the block contract described below, the provider needs to be clear about the shared costs and what funding can be directed by each individual through their ISF.

In the third scenario, ISFs are instigated by providers who have a block contract to provide care for a number of people. This involves the provider disaggregating the overall service budget so that each recipient has an allocated level of funding that is in line with their needs and entitlements. Each person then contributes an element of their individual budget to communal services that they use (including shared support) but individually control the use of the remainder of their budget.

In this book we reflect on the second and third scenarios. We look at the experiences of organisations that have introduced ISFs in order to understand what elements of their change processes were successful and the lessons other organisations have learned from this. We also explore the extent to which ISFs have improved the experiences and opportunities of people accessing their services and the factors that have contributed to positive outcomes being achieved in practice. Earlier learning has already highlighted two key areas for implementing ISFs: the way that the ISF is developed and the relationship with commissioners.

The ISF process

ISFs are essentially an individual budget management process, and whilst they can make an important contribution, this will only lead to positive changes if they are deployed as part of a range of measures seeking to make support more personalised. In other words, simply breaking down the funding available to each service recipient and giving them theoretical power over how this is spent will not work unless the person is supported to both understand their allocation and to make meaningful decisions over how it is used. Due to the disempowerment and lack of information that many people who use services experience, this can be a daunting process for anyone, but even more so for those with whom others find difficulty in communicating and/or those who do not have the capacity to make decisions over all aspects of their lives. What is required is a person-centred process which guides the person through the different stages of the ISF's development and which uses recognised person-centred thinking tools and practices to engage people throughout the process (Figure 1.3).

Developing Individual Service Funds

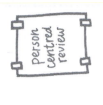

allocation

We look at what your service costs.

We divide this into 'core' money and 'individual' money. The core money is what it costs to deliver your basic service.

The individual money is for you to decide how to spend.

You can have your individual money as individual staff hours if you want.

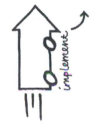

plan

We work with you to develop a plan.

This plan describes what is important to you, how you want to be supported and what you want to achieve in the next year.

The plan will show how you want to use your individual money

agree plan and contract

We put how much individual money you have and how you want to spend this into an agreement or contract.

This means we are accountable to you in how your money is spent.

implement

We use your plan and turn it into a personal weekly plan.

You choose who you want to support you.

We work with you to achieve the goals you set in your plan.

We support you to spend your individual money in the way you want.

ongoing learning

We keep talking to you about how your week and plans are going.

We change things if needed to make sure we get it right for you.

person centred review

We meet together to review your plan and how we are making things happen for you.

We listen to what is working and not working for you.

We tell you how your money is being spent and see if you want to make changes to this.

We look at the goals you put in your plan and what has been achieved.

You say what you want to achieve in the next year and we agree actions to make sure this happens.

Figure 1.3 The Individual Service Fund process (from Sanderson et al.)[7]

7   Sanderson et al. (2012).

The ISF process mirrors the process for developing personal budgets – starting with an upfront allocation of resources (which could be in money or hours). The next step is to develop a support plan to decide what the person wants to change in their life, and what they want their life and week to look like, and this includes how they want to 'spend' their allocation. This plan is then agreed and recorded, then implemented. The implementation results in further learning, and then the allocation, support plan and, most importantly, the impact of all of this on the person's life, is reviewed through a person-centred review. (In Chapters 3–5 we explore this process in detail, using examples and stories from people supported by the organisations.)

The relationship with commissioners

It is now expected practice in social care, and emerging practice in health care, for people who use services to be supported to manage their own budgets. Over time, as society becomes more familiar and confident with these options, this may mean that the majority of individuals eligible for public funding either contract directly with providers and/or employ their own staff; however, in the short term, the local authority or NHS body still holds the personal budget on behalf of most people, and there will probably always be a proportion of people who are unwilling or unable to manage their budget directly. This means that for the foreseeable future, public-sector commissioners are likely to still have a central role in selecting and contracting with providers on behalf of many people. They will continue to be in a powerful position in dictating both what and how support is delivered and therefore a major influence over the development of ISFs. A UK Department of Health's review[8] noted the importance of a collaborative relationship between commissioners and providers if personalisation is going to be taken forward.

Conclusion

Whatever the starting point regarding the funding and care arrangements that are in place, there is the potential opportunity for ISFs to be implemented within services. Whilst the key principles behind ISFs are straightforward and ones that most people in social care will be able to endorse, applying them in practice can seem complicated and difficult in congregate and block funded services. In Chapter 2 we learn about how the organisations have approached the first stage of implementing ISFs – allocating the funding or support hours.

---

8   Bennett and Miller (2009).

Chapter 2

Allocation of Funding

Introduction

The first step to create an ISF is to allocate the funding. In Chapter 1 we introduced three starting points for allocation, and in this chapter we explain how the organisations approached deconstructing block contracts into individual allocations. We have grouped these into 'pure', 'pragmatic' and 'post-planning' approaches. We discuss two common resource allocation tools that are used: the Care Funding Calculator and the Resource Allocation System. Finally, we explore learning from the organisations in relation to the allocation of funding, that is, how this requires financial capacity and ideally support from care managers and commissioners.

Starting points

As outlined in Chapter 1, there are three common starting points in the UK from which ISFs can be developed. These starting points are often connected with particular types of services and management arrangements. Each of these funding arrangements also has implications for providers in relation to the financial sustainability of their services (see Table 2.1); therefore, it is helpful to explain them before looking at what they mean in relation to allocating funding for ISFs.

SPOT-PURCHASED AND INDIVIDUAL PROVISION

The first scenario is an individual spot-purchased package in which the funding available to the individual is clear before the service begins and continues to be managed as such by the provider. If the person using the service decides to receive support from a different provider or to use the funding to meet their desired outcomes in a different way, this funding would follow them. The provider would use the resources for this service to deliver packages to other individuals or cease to provide such a service. The funding for such packages could be through a managed budget held by the purchaser, a direct payment held by the person using the service or their circle of support, or someone paying for a service out of their own resources. Such models are commonly applied in home-care packages and individual tenancies.

SPOT-PURCHASED AND CONGREGATE PROVISION

The second scenario is an individual spot-purchased package in which the funding available to the individual is clear before their service begins, but the provider pools their individual contributions to provide a service to a number of people. The funding provided by each individual is not linked to the level or type of service provided to them in comparison with their peers. If a person decides to go elsewhere, the funding attached to them will be withdrawn and the provider will seek another person to purchase this service. Funding could be through the same sources as in the first scenario, and such models are typically being used in day care, supported employment services and residential care homes.

BLOCK PURCHASED

The third scenario is a block contract arrangement in which a sum of money is given to support a set number of people (e.g. provide a home for six people) and/or deliver a level of service (e.g. up to a set number of hours per week). Funding for such a service comes directly from a public-sector purchaser who identifies which individuals will receive this support and how much of the service will be required by each individual (e.g. days at a centre, number of hours of home care, length of stay in a care home). If someone stops using the service, the funding will remain with the provider and an alternative recipient will be found by the purchaser. This model has been commonly used in local authority day centres, care homes developed through hospital closures and grants to third-sector organisations. This model could also be said to apply to charities that raise funding for direct services through charitable activities, although they are effectively acting as purchaser and provider. There are hybrid models also, for example, if individual support hours are purchased above a block contract due to an individual developing a complex need that would not be covered by the current resources.

Table 2.1 *Different starting points and characteristics*

Scenario	Purchasing arrangement	Common service examples	Extent to which funding within provider is individualised	Funding on exit
1	Individual spot-purchased service	Home-care package Individual-supported tenancy	Funding connected with each individual can be identified. The service directly correlates to level of funding.	Follows the individual
2	Individual spot-purchased service	Independent-sector day care Residential care homes, short-break service, assessment and treatment service	Funding from each individual is pooled to run a congregate service; no individualisation unless the person has identified one-to-one hours.	Follows the individual
3	Block-purchased service	Residential care as part of campus closure Local Authority Day Care	Funding is used to deliver required level and type of service; no individualisation unless the person has identified one-to-one hours additional to block.	Remains with the service (apart from one-to-one hours)

Although it is by no means guaranteed that the funding will be used to promote a personalised response, it is clearly easier to identify and maintain individual funding allocations within scenario 1 (see example of United Response in Box 2.1 for how this can be achieved). In this chapter we therefore explore the processes that have been applied by the organisations within scenarios 2 and 3 to calculate and separate out ISFs.

Box 2.1 ISFs and personal budgets: United Response's approach

United Response supports six people who hold their own personal budget but need support to manage their money. The local authority pays the personal budgets into a special bank account which United Response has opened in order to ensure that these funds are separated from other people's funding. United Response works with the individuals to identify potential community resources that the individuals could use and/or agencies from which they could buy an aspect of their support package. United Response pays the invoices for the support provided, both direct and by another provider. An accessible statement is produced on a monthly basis so that the individuals can see exactly how their money has been spent and what the balance is. United Response levies a small charge for this service.

Here are way United Response supported people to manage their budget in this way:

- One person goes to a very small independent group to do stage acting, singing and dancing. This group is not set up to receive payments directly from the local authority and deals only with cheques and invoices. We are able to pay this so that the person can go to the group.

- One person is helped to ensure they are paying support bills, without this they would have likely gambled all of their money. We manage his ISF and ensure he balances the need to pay for support with his care needs whilst still doing what is important to his overall quality of life – i.e., going out and having the occasional bet.

Pure, post-planning or pragmatic approaches to allocating funding

Organisations have found allocating funding from block contracts to be a complex and time-consuming process, particularly when it is being attempted for the first time. Organisations often told us that they had started with one approach and then had to adapt or switch to a different one when the initial figures did not relate sufficiently to the needs of the individuals and/or the budget available. There were examples of bespoke frameworks being developed and then abandoned, and established tools being used and then adapted (Box 2.2). Based on the experiences of what the organisations described as having worked in practice, we have identified three different approaches that they were able to implement: pure (i.e. identifying resources based on the individual's entitlements); post-planning (i.e. developing a person-centred support plan with the individual and then identifying the resources required to deliver the required support); and pragmatic (i.e. the proportion of the funding within the service that can be freed up from shared costs is divided between people accessing the service).

> ## Box 2.2 One manager's experience of separating out the ISF
>
> One service manager stated:
>
> > We started with a 'rough and ready' approach and used our knowledge of people's support needs to divide the budget amongst all the people on the contract. It was a crude start and not person-centred. The next step was that we devised a matrix to divide people up into different categories depending on their level of need. This caused problems because it was categorising people rather than being person-centred, so we abandoned that approach too.

PURE: THE EXAMPLE OF DIMENSIONS AND REAL LIFE OPTIONS

Dimensions was seeking to apply three key principles of simplicity, transparency and reasonableness, and identified three tests to be used within the funding allocation:

- Each person pays an equal share of the 'core costs' and of any 'shared costs' they require.

- Each person has choice and control over how their 'in-my-personal-control funding' is spent, including the freedom to spend it with another provider.

- If a person leaves the service, the budget (including staff) can be reduced immediately by the value of his or her discretionary funding.

Dimensions' starting point was to develop a means of allocating the existing funding fairly, and the organisation decided to trial two existing tools: the Care Funding Calculator and the Resource Allocation System tool from In Control. Dimensions' intention was to use the two methodologies and then determine the most appropriate tool to use. Unexpectedly, the tools resulted in widely different allocations for everyone. Dimensions' review led the organisation to conclude that these differences were most likely because each tool attempts to measure the same things, but from very different perspectives. Dimensions concluded that the Care Funding Calculator allocation gave a much better reflection of what support people needed and the support they were getting day-to-day. The project manager within Real Life Options used the Care Funding Calculator to identify the support requirements and related budget of the individuals living in the care homes. This was available as a number of support hours for people to use to develop their support plan.

POST-PLANNING: THE EXAMPLE OF CHOICE SUPPORT

Choice Support began by identifying the important people in the person's life (their circle) and implemented a plan. The organisation developed an individual support package based on the plan which outlined the number of hours each person needed. This included one-to-one support and shared hours based on the service in which the person was living at the time. As part of the project, an independent advocate was funded, and she provided comments on all the support plans that were developed (based on person-centred plans) and their associated resource requirements. The completed support plans were then presented to a special panel which consisted of commissioners, care managers and Choice Support representatives. The plans were carefully scrutinised and subject to alterations. For example, support was agreed only for activities that the commissioners viewed as a necessity. The final ISFs were approved by this panel.

PRAGMATIC: THE EXAMPLES OF BRUCE LODGE, CERTITUDE AND LOOK AHEAD

The Bruce Lodge leadership team did not try to deconstruct the block contract into individual budget allocations. They saw this as important for the future, but they decided to begin by identifying how many hours could realistically be under each person's personal control within the staffing complement at that time. This led to a 'budget' of two hours of support per month per person being agreed. Bruce Lodge subsequently further disaggregated the activities budget to identify additional funding connected with each individual resident on top of these personal hours.

Certitude used the Care Funding Calculator in a 'desktop' process to identify how support hours were being used by individuals, providing a breakdown of 'core' and 'flexi' support hours for each person. The calculations from the exercise were then tested over a set period to confirm or adjust the figures. On average, the budget available to each person which would not be part of the shared costs equated to around six hours of support per week in the learning disability services; these were called 'personal control' hours. Personal control hours for people supported in the mental health services varied widely, so Certitude decided that for this prototype stage each resident would have four hours per week of support over which they could have personal control. They focused on hours rather than budget as this was thought to be an easier 'currency' for staff and residents to relate to than the actual financial value. In their pilot at Coventry Road, Look Ahead identified the staffing requirements to meet the core standards of the service in relation to maintaining the welfare and safety of the tenants and the staff (Table 2.2). This accounted for 75 per cent of the budget. The remainder was divided up evenly between the individual tenants to provide them with support hours that they could direct and a 'cash' allocation that could be used flexibly to facilitate access to community resources or purchase items that would improve their quality of life. The funding for the cash was identified through freezing of staffing vacancies. In the rehabilitation service, £35 per week has been built into the budget as a personal allocation for each customer to use to achieve their personal goals.

Table 2.2 *Division of budget in Look Ahead's Coventry Road trial*[1]

Element	Proportion of contract value (%)	What did this cover?
Core	74	Funding was provided for two staff to be on duty at all times to provide routine care and respond to emergencies.
Flexi: cash allocation	8	Each tenant had £40 each week to fund activities or purchase personal items.
Flexi: support hours	18	Each tenant was entitled to 3.5 hours of one-to-one support above the core support to be delivered at a time of their choosing.

1   Table 2.2 is adapted from Look Ahead (2010) *Choice, Control and Independence: Personalising Block Contracts in Supported Housing.* London: Look Ahead.

As you can see, there are two established processes that organisations used to calculate individual allocations. Below is a more detailed exploration of both of them.

Care Funding Calculator

The Care Funding Calculator was developed by the Regional Improvement and Efficiency Partnerships in England. Its primary aim is to help providers and purchasers negotiate a fair price for residential care placements and supported-living packages (Box 2.3). It has been promoted by local authorities as a means to get better value in their purchasing of care services, with estimates that it provided £45 million of savings from such budgets across 51 local authorities between 2008 and 2012. It has also received a degree of support from some providers, such as the Voluntary Organisations Disability Group, as a means to begin discussions on costs of a placement; however, there have also been concerns by providers in relation to some of its methodologies and underlying assumptions. The Care Funding Calculator is seen to be suitable for developing packages for people with a learning disability, mental health and/or physical disabilities, but not for older people. This is because there are different expectations on the models of care provided to older people.

Box 2.3 Aim of the Care Funding Calculator

The aim of the Care Funding Calculator is as follows:

- assess in detail the level of staff support required to meet an individual's needs

- determine a price which is appropriate to the needs of the person and represents the best value for that care based on relevant market knowledge

- confirm any specific outcomes which you have agreed with the service user where they want to develop their skills, and record how this is to be achieved.

(From iESE)[2]

The Care Funding Calculator is based on an Excel spreadsheet which can be downloaded at a charge of £995 per year. The person completing it (who is often a local authority care manager) should work with the person who will receive the support, their family and existing services to complete an assessment of their care and support needs. This includes core aspects of their quality of life such as keeping clean, nourished and safe, and higher aspects such as social contact and meaningful activities. It also considers areas of their life in which the person wants to increase their abilities. The level of support that the person requires for these aspects of care is inputted into the spreadsheet information. This includes considerable detail of their support requirements, including the frequency and duration, the number of staff and the necessary skill levels. The information in the spreadsheet regarding the person's support details is then used to develop a cost model of what funding will be required. The cost model incorporates characteristics of the home such as its location (as there is variation in the cost of living and property prices between areas) and the number of people it will be supporting (as the fixed costs vary depending on the size of service). The Care Funding Calculator then provides a price range as to what it deems a reasonable price for such a service to provide that level of support. Using the Care Funding

---

2   iESE (2013) Care Funding Calculator. The Care Funding Calculator spreadsheet can be downloaded at www.socialcare. improvementefficiency.org.uk/site/cms/contentChapterView.asp?chapter=84, accessed on 12 June 2014.

Calculator to identify the ISF that a person will receive is therefore not the purpose for which the tool was initially developed; however, based on the experiences of the organisations, it can be an informative approach to adopt within the ISF allocation process.

In Control's Resource Allocation System

In Control began work on producing a better system to allocate social care resources in 2003. The organisation built upon previous experience of the introduction of more individualised funding in the closure of a long-stay hospital in Scotland, and over the years it has produced five versions of its Resource Allocation System. This was developed initially in collaboration with local authority adult social service developments but has also been applied within children's services.

The core principles behind the Resource Allocation System are as follows:

- *Transparency*. Everyone knows what is happening, the basis for decisions being made and no decisions are taken 'behind closed doors'.

- *Participation*. All those who need to be involved, including the individual and their family, are involved and their views lead the discussion.

The process involves people who currently access, and who subsequently enter, services upon completing a self-assessment questionnaire. This is a simple questionnaire that measures and scores the impact of a person's disability on their life in a number of key areas. The impact scores of each are added up, and then the total score is adjusted according to the level and type of support that is reasonably available to that person from their friends and families. So someone with a strong network of support will have a lower final score than someone with the same impact of disability without any informal support. Funding is allocated on the basis of this score, the agreed outcomes that the person and their family want to achieve and the typical costs of achieving these outcomes in the local area. (The latter is calculated from analysis of people currently receiving support and the costs that are currently associated with their care.)

In Control emphasises that whilst this process is helpful to give an initial framework of funding, it should be seen as the starting point rather than the end point. For example, once the system has been in operation for some time, the experiences of people who have their own personal budget can be drawn upon to review the funding connected with meeting different outcomes rather than relying solely on data from the previous funding system. In Control also stresses that whilst figures from other areas that use Resource Allocation Systems may be helpful to learn from, it is vital that each one reflect the local context. This requires active and ongoing involvement in the development and review of the system by people who use services, their families, care professionals, managers and finance departments. Finally, In Control suggests a number of criteria which can be used to assess the strength of a Resource Allocation System (Table 2.3).

In Control is working with providers to further develop the Resource Allocation System to assist both providers and commissioners in deconstructing block contracts into ISF allocations. Whichever approach an organisation used, there were three other factors that had an impact on how the allocations were reached: finance capacity and skills, maximising the funding available for ISFs, and support from commissioners and care managers.[3]

---

3   For further information regarding the In Control Resource Allocation System, see www.in-control.org.uk/support/support-for-organisations/resource-allocation-systems-(ras).aspx.

Table 2.3 *Criteria to assess a Resource Allocation System*[4]

Aspect	Outcome
Transparency	The RAS methodology must be in the public domain at a community level.
Simplicity	The process must be simple and the individual and their family must know how the decision was reached for them.
Sufficiency	The council must publish clearly the outcomes they will enable people to achieve and the support put in place must be enough to reasonably achieve these.
Control	The person must know the amount of money in their budget as early as possible in the process and be able to use the budget in ways and at times of their choosing to achieve agreed outcomes.

Three factors impacting how allocations were reached

FINANCE CAPACITY AND SKILLS

Certitude had previously calculated the support available to each individual, but this had become overly complicated and therefore had not been implemented in practice. Building on this experience, it was recognised that the contribution of the finance team would be vital, and therefore a dedicated personalisation accountant post was created. This person was responsible for providing hands-on support to the project to enable managers to understand how to break down their support hours and to work with the director of finance to consider implications for accounting approaches and systems. The personalisation accountant undertook a series of briefings for staff within the services regarding ISFs and the Care Funding Calculator, and also acted as a contact point for queries.

MAXIMISING THE FUNDING AVAILABLE FOR ISFS

Before embarking on the development of ISFs, Choice Support undertook a number of cost-saving initiatives. These initiatives were to ensure that the organisation could be confident that this funding would be sustained in the future and that as much of the funding as possible would be available for direct care. Costs were reduced through:

- reducing the unit hourly costs of direct care by streamlining the management structure and changing staff terms and conditions

- ensuring that overheads were kept to a maximum of 15 per cent by, for example, closing the local office

- using telecare as an alternative to direct care, particularly during waking-night support

- de-registering care home to tenancies with support.

---

4   See www.in-control.org.uk/what-we-do/children-and-young-people/useful-resources/resource-allocation-systems-(ras). aspx for more information.

SUPPORT FROM COMMISSIONERS AND CARE MANAGERS

The organisations have had mixed experiences of engagement with commissioners and/or care managers. In the examples of Choice Support and Look Ahead's rehabilitation service, there was strong support from the local authority and NHS, and this provided a degree of certainty regarding the continuation of the funding for the services and the ISFs available for individuals. Care managers and commissioners also provided helpful alternative perspectives regarding the support needs of the individual and different approaches to meeting these needs; however, when there was a lack of engagement, then the opposite was true, with providers either perceiving (or being told) that ISFs were no longer a priority for the local authority or that their calculations of the funding available were not correct or indeed legitimate.

As you can see, the organisations we learned from tried a variety of approaches to working out the allocations for individuals as the first part of developing an ISF. The organisations that were committed to identifying an allocation before planning (the 'pure' approach) experimented with the Care Funding Calculator and the Resource Allocation System. Another organisation allocated the funding based on person-centred planning (the 'post-planning' approach) which, it could be argued, is closer to a good care management process, where the plan determines the funding rather than the funding being allocated before planning. The third approach was a pragmatic allocation before planning, but without an allocation based on need. This approach was taken by organisations as a starting place to introduce the principles of ISF, where there is an upfront allocation and then people are supported to plan how to use this allocation.

Whatever approach they took to separating out the funding the organisations all needed considerable tenacity to overcome the various barriers and uncertainties that they encountered. Dimensions reflect on their experience as follows:

> It is true that the money issue is often a thorny one, and one that can have people with considerable experience scratching their heads. We needed to face the probability that the conversations, figures, processes and pressures would vary from person to person, but that our sole aim had to be finding the amount that was in a person's personal control. We're now committed to that.

This is the most important issue in relation to allocation – that people know how much money is in their personal control.

Conclusion

When we are setting up new services it is relatively easy to start on the basis that people should have the funding available to them clearly identified and for accountability mechanisms regarding their use to be built around their wishes. For services that are already in existence, particularly those in congregate settings and with block contracts this is a more complex undertaking. In this chapter we have learned how the organisations have sought to untangle existing processes and budget and at least begin the journey towards providing full ISFs. This requires considerable tenacity, a willingness to sort out problems that arise and a commitment from the finance department along with operational managers. Tools such as the Care Funding Calculator and the Resource Allocation System can provide a structure to the process and a means to begin the discussion about who is entitled to what level of funding. Support from key stakeholders outside of the organisation such as commissioners and care managers are also key.

In Chapter 3 we consider how the organisations have supported individuals to think about how they want to use this funding and support to live their life, with as much choice and control over these decisions as possible.

Chapter 3
Planning

Introduction

Once an individual knows what their allocation is, the next part of the ISF process is to think about how they want to use their budget to live their life. This is done through support planning. In Chapter 2 we looked at the different ways that organisations approached the allocation of funding; however this is done, it is the sequence that is important, so that people know how much money they have in their personal control before they start to plan.

Good support planning is an opportunity to think and reflect, explore options and decide which ones could work best. The majority of the organisations we looked at used a support planning process based on a meeting, and others developed support plans with people using person-centred thinking tools, on a one-to-one basis.

In this chapter we start by looking at the information that needs to be in a support plan, then look at different ways that this can be gathered through person-centred thinking and planning, and through meeting-based processes such as Planning Live and one-page profile meetings. It is easy for support planning to be reduced to completing a set of paperwork, however 'person-centred' that paperwork may be. Finally, we look at how this information can be recorded in the support plan.

Information required for a good support plan

Early work around support planning by In Control identified seven criteria by which to judge support plans. In 2012, Think Local Act Personal produced guidance on support planning which recommends that a support plan summary be signed off at the local authority level, without needing to see the detail of the support plan in order to agree the funding. Within the implementation of personal budgets, there have been concerns about the length of support plans and ensuring that they are proportionate to the level of funding being agreed.

It is important to go back to the purpose of support planning within the context of an ISF. The purpose of the planning is to enable people to reflect on what matters to them, where they want to be in the future (their outcomes) and how they plan to use their budget to achieve their outcomes. The support plan therefore is the blueprint of the service design and delivery that the person will expect from their provider. Because of this, it is vital that the support plan have the detail of what matters to the person, what this means for their support, the outcomes that they are seeking and the day-to-day detail of what good support means to them; thus, in support planning within an ISF context, it would not be possible to enable people to be supported to have choice and control over their life and service without a plan that describes how they want to live, and therefore we return to the original seven criteria developed by In Control,[1] slightly modified to relate to ISFs. These criteria are as follows:

1. What is important to you?

   If someone reads the plan, they should get a good sense of the real you. They should get an understanding of what matters to you, your personality, interests and hopes for the future.

---

1   For more information, see www.in-control.org.uk/resources/support-planning.aspx, accessed 16 June 2014.

2. What do you want to change?

The plan should state what you want to change about your life. This may include changing where you live, changing how you are supported or changing how you spend your time. These are your outcomes – how you want your life to be different in a year's time.

3. How will you be supported?

The plan should state what kind of support you want and need to live your life. It should state how you will make sure that you stay safe and well.

4. How will you spend your personal budget?

The plan must set out what the support service will cost for a year – how you will use your hours or money to live your life and make the changes that you want to see over the next year.

5. How will your support be managed?

The plan must explain how any support you pay for is going to be organised. This could include who you want to support you.

6. How will you stay in control of your life?

The plan must say how you will stay in control of your own life. This means looking at what decisions you make, and when other people make decisions for you, how they make sure that you are involved and that you agree to them.

7. What are you going to do to make this plan happen (action plan)?

The plan should set out real and measurable things that will have happened in the future so that it is possible to see whether or not the plan is working.

It is also very important that support plans have contingency plans, particularly when people have a fluctuating long-term health or mental health condition.

Person-centred thinking, person-centred planning and support planning

Great support planning reflects a person-centred ethos; however, support planning is different to person-centred planning. The first difference is that support planning begins with an individual indicative allocation of money, and the purpose is to support people to think about how they want to spend this to achieve the life that they want. Person-centred planning is a term that refers to a family of approaches that focus on how the person wants to live now, and a vision for their future. Person-centred planning results in actions to move towards that future, and this may include seeking funding. In support planning, this funding is allocated up front, before the person starts to plan.

This is an important principle in support planning, as the allocation has an impact on decision-making. For example, if you are planning a holiday, one of the first considerations is likely to be how much you can afford to spend. If it is a few hundred pounds, you may be looking at camping or a house swap. If your budget is significantly bigger, you may be looking at a holiday abroad for a couple of weeks. It would be unusual to plan your holiday without having an indication of how much you have to spend.

Many people use person-centred planning and thinking as the foundation of support planning. They started with an allocation and then used person-centred planning or person-centred thinking tools to think about their life, make decisions and record that in the support plan. Organisations can either use person-centred planning as the basis of support planning, as Look Ahead did, or use existing person-centred plans to inform support planning, as Imagine, Act and Succeed (IAS) did. Even when these organisations used person-centred planning, the allocation was still made before using this information for support planning. The staff at Look Ahead had training in person-centred thinking and planning so that they would be able to assist people in developing their support plans, if required. Once the allocation was agreed, Look Ahead gave people they support the opportunity to have an externally facilitated person-centred plan as the basis of their support plan. In the early phase of developing ISFs, 19 out of 20 people used person-centred thinking and planning in their support plans. The review of the Look Ahead project on ISFs found that one of the keys to the success of their model was the facilitated person-centred planning that underpinned customers' support plans.

Some people may already have a person-centred plan, and the allocation and support plan builds on this information. This is what happened for Paul, who is supported by IAS, which is working on formalising many of the arrangements that have evolved. IAS has experimented with ways of putting more choice and control into people's hands using the principles of ISFs.

Paul's story

Paul moved from a long-stay institution into a shared tenancy for four people in 1994. He was on a Home Office section and this acted to curb any thoughts about other possibilities. Paul was aware of other people moving on from the 'group home' model, and he began to talk about his aspirations and dreams. Paul invited key people in his life to help him create a PATH, and this person-centred planning revealed, amongst other things, that Paul 'wanted freedom'. Paul had been supported to dream, and his vision of an ideal life encouraged the IAS to overcome many obstacles. Paul moved into his own two-bed terraced house two years after his PATH meeting and ten years after moving back to Wigan. As explained by Ruth Gorman, CEO and then head of operations at IAS:

> Really working in partnership from a shared set of values, and jointly figuring out how to make things happen, has been at the heart of our work in Wigan. We looked at the resource being used for four people and worked out how it could be better used to support 'three plus one' people. Paul took 30 hours of contact time from the allocation of 210 hours with the remaining 180 hours providing the right level of support for the other three people.

Paul got the support needed for his life, and the three men benefited from an improved living environment. The Housing Association played their part in reconfiguring the rents to make it all stack up. Paul had an allocation of 30 hours, and we used his PATH to inform his support plan, and to help him to move.

> Paul became a little anxious close to moving to his own place. It would have been easy to put a brake on the move and to have kept Paul in the protective environment of a group home.

To get through this difficult time, Paul didn't need wrapping in cotton wool – he needed support, as most people do when facing a challenge. Natural tendencies to (over) protect a vulnerable person can get in the way of recognising and developing a person's capacity. 'Person-centred working is about getting alongside a person, working through the anxieties and going at their pace,' Ruth continues.

Paul has a very different lifestyle now, with an expanded range of friends and acquaintances. Likewise, he has a very different relationship with the staff that supports him. He can decide:

- when he is supported
- by whom he is supported
- whether he wants all 30 hours in a particular week.

Paul monitors the use of his 30 hours with his team leader and they keep a running total of hours used and therefore a balance. Paul loves to travel. When he's in unfamiliar places, he needs greater support. He can plan a 'city break' by saving up the additional hours he'll need. Paul is one example where IAS has managed to identify the resource a person is allocated, to ring-fence it for that person's support and to work in person-centred ways to enable the individual to have real choice and control over their lives through creating an ISF.

HOW PERSON-CENTRED PLANS CAN CONTRIBUTE TO SUPPORT PLANS

Below are some of the commonly used styles of person-centred planning and how they contribute information to a support plan.

PATH

Regarding PATH, you will have the following information:

- what the person wants to change and move towards (positive and possible, i.e. 'north star')
- who the key people are in the person's life.

You will need to develop the following information:

- what is important to the person
- how they need to be supported
- how they will spend their individual budget and manage their support
- how they will stay in control of their life
- an action plan.

Essential Lifestyle Plan

Regarding the Essential Lifestyle Plan, you will have the following information:

- what and who is important to the person
- what good support looks like
- how the person communicates
- what is working and not working for the person at the moment.

You will need to develop the following information:

- what the person wants for the future
- how they will spend their individual budget and manage their support

- how they will stay in control of their life

- an action plan.

Personal Futures Plan

Regarding the Personal Futures Plan, you will have the following information:

- where the person goes in the community now

- what support they want and need

- who the important people are in their life

- what their dreams are.

You will need to develop the following information:

- what is important to the person

- how they will spend their individual budget and manage their support

- how they will stay in control of their life

- an action plan.

Jennie's story

When people have families or a circle of support around them, they are likely to be very involved in developing the support plan with the person. Jennie has an ISF with provider Independent Options. Suzie, Jennie's mother, and the circle of support used developed Jennie's support plan with her based on existing person-centred plans. Suzie states:

> We had 80 per cent of the information we needed for Jennie's support plan from her Essential Lifestyle Plan and PATH. Jennie's Essential Lifestyle Plan had all the information about what was important to Jennie and the support that she needed on a day-to-day basis. The PATH captured our hopes and dreams for the future. We based our decision on this, our collective understanding of Jennie. Whilst we decided to get extra help to think about Jennie's future home, we knew that we could put her 'perfect week' together in a meeting with her circle of support.
>
> As well as what Jennie may want to do during her week (for her perfect week), we also wanted to include how she stays in touch with the people who are important to her, and how and when she develops her friendships. Once we identified a range of interests, places and hobbies that are important to Jennie, and the relationships that are important to her, we looked at how we could incorporate them into a perfect week. We took an A4 sheet of paper and wrote Monday to Sunday across the top and then 'morning', 'lunch', 'afternoon', 'tea' and 'evening' down the side. Then we slotted all the activities into a perfect week for Jennie, including a college course (art, music), dance class, going to the gym, horse riding, swimming and Jacuzzi, cinema, bowling, trampolining, going to the pub for tea, spending time with family, seeing her friends, relaxing at home listening to music, being creative and watching DVDs. Obviously this was more than she could do in one week, so this extended into her 'perfect month'. We added up what it would cost for Jennie to have a cinema card, entrance to a gym, classes, entrance to bowling and so on, to see what she would need each week.
>
> We also used her PATH to inform Jennie's perfect week by keeping in mind our ultimate goal of what Jennie's future should look like. This was how we went from the

Essential Lifestyle Plan to the PATH, to the community map to the perfect week – and this trail of person-centred planning and thinking tools all ended up being incorporated into the support plan.

HOW PERSON-CENTRED THINKING TOOLS CAN CONTRIBUTE TO SUPPORT PLANS

Usually in support planning people start by thinking about their life and what they want to change, and then how they want to make these changes with their money, resources, skills and connections. Once the person knows what they want to change and what resources they have to make that change, the next step is to come up with options and ideas. From this list of ideas, people can make final decisions about how they want to live their life and use their budget, and this is recorded in their support plan.

There are person-centred thinking tools that can help with each of these steps. You can use any or all of them. You do not need to use all of them in each section; you can just choose the one you like the best, or do two or three if you want. Figure 3.1 shows the range of person-centred thinking tools that directly contribute to the information required for a good, detailed support plan.

It is crucial that the support plan not be a new form to complete or a new tick box for an organisation to achieve. The support plan determines how the service is delivered, and therefore it should have an impact on who and how the person is supported, exactly what they do each week, and how the staff are supported, coached and supervised, down to what is discussed within team meetings. This is described in later chapters, and Jenny's story (note the spelling difference as compared with 'Jennie', who is another person) shows how the person-centred thinking tools used within her support plan make a day-to-day difference in her life.

Jenny's story

Jenny is supported by Certitude, and Shaun Lindley, who manages Jenny's service and ISF, describes the person-centred thinking tools used within Jenny's support plan and how using these tools is making a difference in her life:

Jenny is 43 years old and is a very likeable, intelligent, witty and kind person. She has a 20-year history of serious mental health issues including long periods spent in hospital. Her various diagnoses of schizoaffective disorder, bipolar affective disorder, hypomania and hysterical fugue have manifested themselves in significant symptoms including several suicide attempts, regular self-harming, setting light to her hair and swallowing glass.

When Jenny first came to one of Certitude's registered mental health services in London two years ago, there were some questions as to whether she could cope with living in a community setting. This was due in part to the fact that it can be difficult to find successful ways to motivate and encourage Jenny to take part in activities outside of the home.

Jenny has serious and enduring mental health issues. Her major self-esteem issues mean that she considers herself to be evil, useless and ugly, and she believes that everyone dislikes her. She spends long periods of time isolated in her room not wanting contact with anyone, feeling scared and anxious. Jenny is scared of bathing and her personal care can suffer as a result.

The person-centred thinking tools that were part of Jenny's support plan include Relationship Circles, Perfect Week, Matching, Decision-making Agreement and Working/Not Working, and these tools soon began to show positive results.

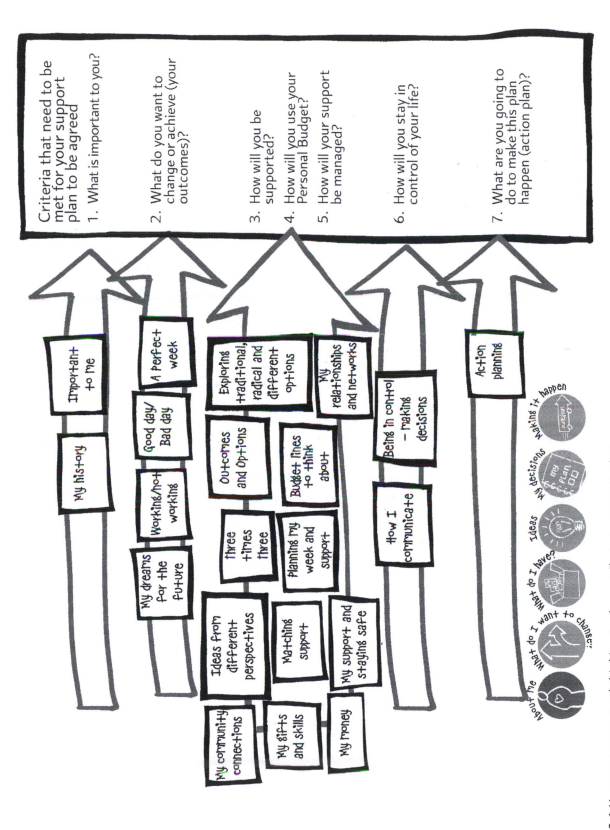

Criteria that need to be met for your support plan to be agreed

1. What is important to you?

2. What do you want to change or achieve (your outcomes)?

3. How will you be supported?

4. How will you use your Personal Budget?

5. How will your support be managed?

6. How will you stay in control of your life?

7. What are you going to do to make this plan happen (action plan)?

Important to me

A perfect week

Exploring traditional, radical and different options

My relationships and networks

Action planning

My history

Good day/ Bad day

Outcomes and options

Budget lines to think about

Being in control – making decisions

Working/not working

three times three

Planning my week and support

How I communicate

My dreams for the future

Ideas from different perspectives

Matching support

My support and staying safe

My community connections

My gifts and skills

My money

About me

What do I want to change?

What do I have?

Ideas

My decisions my plan

Making it happen action

Figure 3.1 How person-centred thinking tools contribute to support plans

As well as basing support planning on person-centred planning and person-centred thinking tools, there are meeting-based approaches that use person centred thinking tools to develop a support plan. The first of these approaches is Planning Live.

Planning Live

Planning Live was originally developed to support the UK Department of Health's individual budget pilot sites to move quickly in supporting the first cohort of people to develop their support plans; however, it is a very useful process for bringing people together in the same room to help the person think about their life and put together their support plan.

The Planning Live process can be used either by people who live together in a household, as Real Life Options and Dimensions used it, or by people who live in the same neighbourhood, as Certitude used it, to get started on their support plan. The process usually involves between four and six individuals and the people close to them, and takes place over two consecutive days. The individuals and the people they invite each have their own table and work together, but there are several points of sharing and mutual support throughout the two days.

Carolyn was involved in the first Planning Live that took place in Dimensions, and she states:

> Planning Live really felt like the start of the journey for us all. My staff and I spent two whole days listening – and that's it, just listening to the people we support. We gleaned so much information over those two days which enabled the people we support to think more about how their life was for them and their families. So much was covered in Planning Live.

WHO IS INVOLVED?

Each individual is supported to develop their relationship circle, to think about who is important to him or her and who they want to invite to their Planning Live. This could include family members, circle members, professionals, people who support them in their staff team or advocates. One of the advantages of Planning Live is that if everyone in a household is involved in Planning Live, then the staff team on duty can all be present throughout the process.

Bree's story

Bree, who lives with two other women, invited her boyfriend, social worker and brother to Planning Live. As her brother works, he took the day off to attend the first day. He found it such a powerful experience that he took the second day off work as well in order to attend the full event. Bree's social worker could only attend for two hours at the beginning of the process, but she used these two hours well to share all that she knew about Bree and her life.

Managers play a significant role in Planning Live. They can also be the facilitators. One organisation trained and supported their managers to be able to facilitate the two-day Planning Live sessions. Managers attended a two-day training course to prepare them, then each acted as a 'coach' during a Planning Live that a trainer delivered. They then had the opportunity to co-lead a Planning Live with the trainer, and then started to deliver Planning Live in pairs with another manager. Another organisation developed a new coaching role that includes facilitating Planning Live. This gives a further degree of independence.

What happens in Planning Live?

Michelle, a Planning Live facilitator, supported Bree in Planning Live. Here is how she describes the process:

Within those two days, we used the principles of person-centred thinking to capture rich information, and this helped us think about how we could be using the person's allocation. We started with using the person-centred thinking tool 'working and not working' from different perspectives to get a good understanding of what life is like now for the person. This also helped us to start thinking about the person's outcomes and actions for their future.

One of the things we pay particular attention to with Planning Live is figuring out what a perfect week would look like. When considering what a 'perfect week' actually means, we think about what matters to the person most from a 'worth getting up in the morning for' and 'what makes life worth living' perspective, to how do we keep them healthy and safe within that framework. So it's a perfect, balanced week we're thinking about.

Some of the other person-centred thinking tools that we use are the relationship circle and thinking about the person's connections, so that we can make sure that when we're developing a perfect week, we're thinking about the people who are currently important to the person, or who they'd like to be important in the future.

We also look at the person's community so that we can develop a community map to help think about places they would want to spend their perfect week. We also develop some outcomes we can move towards, such as within a year, what would they like to change or achieve? And how can we put that within their prefect week? We then look at their allocation and think about how we can plan the cost of a perfect week. Not all of a perfect week requires cost, because there may be unpaid or natural resources that help us think about the person's perfect week.

There are basically three elements to Planning Live (Figure 3.2): the preparation; the 'what happens during the workshops'; and the 'what happens after the workshops', where we make sure we've pulled all the information together to create a robust support plan.

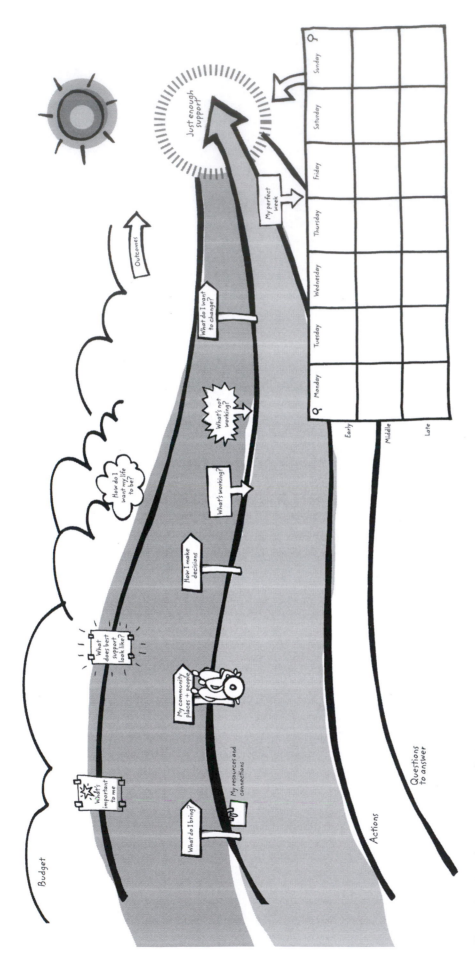

Figure 3.2 Graphic summary of Planning Live

Albert's story: Planning Live

Albert is an elderly man with a learning disability and visual impairment who lives in 24-hour residential care. Due to health issues, he had been on 24-hour bed rest for the past 12 months, and he had not only become withdrawn from his community because he never went out of the house, but was also isolated from the four other people with whom he lives. The only people involved in Albert's life were the district nurses and his staff team. Although his staff team knew he had a fantastic sense of humour and loved a joke, staff reported that even this had deteriorated and Albert rarely spoke about anything apart from the odd grumble.

When the possibility of Albert taking part in the Planning Live workshops was discussed with him and his team, his staff had mixed opinions about the benefits. Most of the staff felt that he would not stay, and that if he came at all, he would ask to go home as soon as he got there. Some staff were more optimistic, believing that even if he stayed for a short time, this would still be positive for Albert as he had gotten used to not going out. Albert did not have any friends or family in his relationship circle; therefore, a key part of the preparation process was to identify the staff in whom Albert had confidence and trusted to support him during the workshops. It was important that he could be supported by staff who could see what was possible for Albert and would encourage him to develop his self-confidence in being out of his home environment. It was obvious from his relationship circles that Albert had become increasingly isolated and had only a few meaningful, paid relationships.

The staff team worked hard on getting prepared for the workshops and had explored what a good day and bad day currently looked like to Albert, and this helped them to develop his one-page profile and he brought this to the workshop along with his communication charts and his staff's draft one-page profiles.

Albert appeared quite tense when he arrived with his staff team and the people with whom he lived to the first day of the Planning Live workshop. The community-based venue had been chosen because it had enough space for five people to take part in Planning Live in the same room, and had great access and space for people to use the gardens if they wanted. Although there was music playing in the background and a welcoming, lively environment, we quickly learned that while this worked for others, it was probably a bit overwhelming for Albert. While staff attempted to settle him into his own separate space within the room, he started to take in his surroundings. Unfortunately, the careful planning that had gone into preparing him to take part came undone when a member of staff who did not know him so well offered him a cup of tea. In most circumstances this would be a perfectly natural thing to do; however, anyone who knows Albert well understands that if you offer him a cup of tea while he is out, he will become anxious and start to ask to go home. This is exactly what happened, and Albert stayed for only ten minutes on the first day. With lessons learned and clear instructions given to staff who did not know him well about what good support looks like to Albert when in the Planning Live environment, Albert returned for the second day. Staff told jokes and indulged in lively banter to ensure that Albert felt happy and relaxed. He even joined in a sing-song when the group was recording things that were working well for Albert around music. Albert was happy to stay for as long as he was physically able, as he can sit in his moulded wheelchair for a maximum of only five hours. Albert exceeded everybody's expectations and demonstrated that, with the right support around him, he could actively participate in planning his own life. This was an important milestone for his team, as by the end of the workshop, they had developed a much richer week that would enable Albert to achieve his outcomes.

From Planning Live we had gathered lots of detailed information from people who cared about Albert and new him well. Although there was already a lot of information recorded about him, much of it was health related and focused on what was important for him. The workshop and Albert's ability to take part had helped his team to see him differently and recognise that there was much more to Albert than his health issues and disability. Everyone's expectations for what his life could look like in comparison with his current reality were raised. Deeper conversations at the workshop resulted in a much better understanding of the things that made Albert's life worth living. Michelle, the team manager, said:

> Albert's team had been so focused on keeping him healthy and safe that they had lost sight of what gave him a good quality of life. Prior to Planning Live, I'd never known Albert to go out socially. Although his health needs are still important, this isn't the sole focus of their support anymore. This has opened them up to trying new things with him and being less risk averse.

KEY ELEMENTS OF THE PROCESS

The outcomes from Planning Live are detailed person-centred information (completed person-centred thinking tools), a summary of how the person wants to live (their 'perfect week') and how they want their life to be different in a year (their personal outcomes). When Dimensions reviewed its initial experience of developing ISFs, the organisation identified the four key elements below for Planning Live.

Independent facilitation and challenge

Planning Live is most powerful when it is facilitated independently. The independent facilitator might be someone who is completely removed from the organisation, or is part of the organisation but not necessarily related to the person or the service. The benefit of this is that there is a degree of challenge that otherwise would not be present. It can be helpful to gently challenge assumptions ('he always needs two staff to do this') and support people to aspire and think creatively about possibilities. The facilitator can challenge any limiting assumptions by asking questions to which people think they already know the answers in a way that feels safe. They can also make sure that they are constantly asking 'Is this right?' because they do not know the person well.

Michelle, a Planning Live facilitator, relates the following:

> When I was facilitating Planning Live for five people who shared their home and support, I was able to spend time with each group checking out any assumptions from the information that was being gathered. One experience that stands out for me was when I introduced myself to one of the women who was developing her plan. She had a group of people around her including family and staff. I noticed that staff were referring to her as either Pat or Pattie, so I asked what she preferred. She paused and said, 'I'd rather be called Patricia'. The staff members looked surprised and asked her why she had never mentioned this before. Patricia responded that no one had asked her before.

Good preparation

Good practical preparation is crucial. The manager and staff who are organising Planning Live need to think about the environment so that it is conducive to clear thinking and planning. There needs to be planning to ensure that people are supported to fully participate. It is crucial that everybody who comes to Planning Live be clear beforehand about the purpose and what their role will be. The logistics are very important: making sure people can get there on time, that there are refreshments, that staff are rostered accordingly to avoid a staff change-over halfway through the day and so forth.

Confidence in using person-centred thinking tools

The more confident and comfortable that staff are in using person-centred thinking tools, the easier the process will be. The person-centred thinking tools that are used in Planning Live are as follows:

- one-page profiles
- working and not working from different perspectives
- relationship circle
- community map
- communication chart
- decision-making agreement
- perfect week.

It is possible to facilitate Planning Live without staff being familiar with these person-centred thinking tools, but it is always a much better process when they are.

Michelle, the Planning Live facilitator quoted above, had this to say:

> One organisation that I worked with was learning about person-centred thinking tools as we held the Planning Live workshops. This didn't get in the way of the planning, but it did mean that participants needed additional support and coaching around understanding some of the person-centred thinking tools. This meant that there was quite a bit of best guessing and testing out when it came to exploring what needed to be in the 'perfect week'. In another organisation, all the staff had been trained and were habitually using person-centred thinking tools and practices. Because of this, the workshops were able to focus on further developing and updating the rich information that they already had and ensured that everyone was confident that the 'perfect week' was a true reflection of how the person really wanted to spend their time.

Getting to a 'perfect week'

Good person-centred planning processes result in much of the information that we need to help people change their life. Planning Live results in a different kind of summary, as it brings together everything that has been learned with the person into their perfect week, and their personal outcomes, as well as detailed person-centred information. The 'perfect week' is not an 'if I win the lottery' perfect week, but rather a perfect week which is within the possibilities of the budget allocation the person has.

To develop the perfect week starts with relationships:

- Who is important in the person's life, and when and where do they want to see and connect with people (using the relationship circle)?
- What is important in the person's life, and when and where do they do this (using the one-page profile)?
- Where does the person go in their community? When do they want to go to these places?
- What support does the person need? When and where does this need to be delivered?

The perfect week balances planning and flexibility. For example, there may be some things that have to happen on a particular day of the week.

Anne-Marie helped Dimensions to learn about ISFs and was the first person to use Planning Live in the organisation. Table 3.1 shows her current perfect week with a balance of what has to happen on a certain day (Church coffee morning) and what is flexible.

Table 3.1 *An example of a perfect week developed through Planning Live*

	Morning	**Afternoon**	**Evening**
Mon	Dog walking (paid employment), 1 hour	Swimming lesson (local pool) followed by café 15:00 to 16:30	
Tue	Working in café, sailing club 10:00 to 12:00 weekly	Armchair exercise group, local GP surgery 14:00 to 15:00	Baking weekly
Wed	Dog walking (paid employment), 1 hour	Visit Dad and Daphne fortnightly	Bead club (local craft group) 19:30 to 21:00
Thu	Advocacy group (Eastleigh) 10:30 to 12:30; followed by lunch out		Cinema with friends monthly or DVD evening
Fri	Food shopping weekly	Visit or have visit from friends or meet up for a drink	Pamper evening every 2 months at local church or weekly at home
Sat	Visit or have visit from friends or meet up for coffee	Voluntary job (charity shop), 2 hours	Takeaway food fortnightly
Sun	Helping in kitchen for Church coffee morning 12:00 to 12:30	See Terry at home, his house or out weekly	Out for a drink in local pub

THE ADVANTAGES OF USING PLANNING LIVE

Four of the main benefits of using Planning Live (i.e. connection, timeliness, contribution, and sharing and building a depth of knowledge about the person and how they want to live) are given below.

Connection

Planning Live gives the person an opportunity to share ideas and experiences with others who are in the same situation, for example, people who live together in the same household. People can hear and learn from other people's experiences, which they can build on by using those ideas as well as their own. Everybody gets the same information at the same time, so everybody feels supported and connected by doing it together.

Billy's story

Billy came to Planning Live to support his sister-in-law, Bernice. At the beginning of the first day he said that he was not sure if he would have much to contribute as the staff knew her really well, but that he was still willing to take part. What quickly became apparent was that Billy had incredible local knowledge and contacts. Every time a new idea about how Bernice might want to spend her time differently was presented, he not only knew a place or organisation where she might be able to do that, he also knew many of the organisers. When each group came together to share their learning and ideas, Billy was also able to make suggestions and link the groups up to people he knew. Billy became the 'go to' person over the two days whenever we needed to discover who or what was in the community.

Timeliness

As stated earlier, Planning Live was originally developed to support the individual budget pilots to meet one of their early deadlines for having 15 people with a support plan. Where there is a sense of urgency to complete support plans, Planning Live is a good way to enable them to be completed over a two-day period (with preparation). Where three or four people live together, developing support plans on a one-to-one basis could take three or four weeks, or sometimes longer. Planning Live means that each person has their support plan developed quickly so that the emphasis can then be placed on implementing, updating and reviewing it. Doing it together also means that when decisions have to be negotiated or agreed with a few people, it can happen there and then.

Bernice, Eva and Dianne's story

When Bernice, Eva and Dianne took part in Planning Live, they had decided to do this in their own home as it was spacious and had enough rooms to enable each of them to plan with their families and support staff. As each group worked together they created their own thinking space and became absorbed in the planning. As the facilitator of the three groups, Michelle encouraged them to take regular opportunities to share reflections, ideas and learning. It was at one of these breaks from the planning that a member of the staff shared that one of the things that had not been working for Bernice was staff coming on shift at 8 a.m. on a Sunday. She had said that she would prefer a Sunday lie-in and did not need staff to be around but would rather have extra staff working in the afternoon so that she could go out for her Sunday dinner. At this point Eva said that was what she had also identified as not working. The manger of the staff team was immediately able to ask Dianne how she felt about this. Dianne said that she thought it was a good idea, so the decision was to change the rotas to enable the women to not only have a lie-in without staff being around but also to move the two saved hours to the afternoon so that going out for a meal would now be immediately possible.

Contribution

As all staff on duty can be part of Planning Live, and often staff who are not on duty also attend (and get time in lieu for this), this means that everyone supporting a person can contribute their information. It also ensures that all staff know what is happening, how the information was developed and can start to see how the support plan can be delivered. In other words, there is a greater sense of connection.

Lilly's story

Lilly is 87 years old and has a hearing impairment. Lilly's staff were apprehensive about Planning Live, that is, they were unsure about whether she would be able to attend the workshops due to her age and a recent period of serious ill health that has left her extremely frail. They also were not sure of what the family would make of her participation, as the planning meetings that they were accustomed to followed a conventional format were people would sit around a table, talk about Lilly and take notes. When her sister and niece arrived, they were introduced to the process and the large visual Planning Live graphic template. Almost immediately Lilly's niece became emotional and explained that this had taken her back to years ago when Lilly was living in an institute and had been involved in some person-centred planning. She said that this had been a time when Lilly had been truly involved in the planning, rather than others making plans for her. She explained that Lilly was a visual person and that this style of planning not only worked best for her, but also enabled her sister, who also has a hearing impairment, to be fully involved. June, the manager of Lilly's service, said that the Planning Live process had enabled Lilly's sister and niece to feel that they could actively contribute to ideas and actions. In particular, they were delighted to have a role in better supporting Lilly to capture her family history. Everyone knew that Lilly already treasured her family photos; however, staff supporting Lilly at the workshop shared that they had only a limited amount of historical information about Lilly, that the only photos she had were quite recent and that they would value learning more about Lilly's history and past relationships.

Lilly's sister suggested that they create a 'memory box' and find photos of Lilly in her youth and people she has known through the years so that family and staff would be able to look through these photos with Lilly and celebrate her life and experiences. Gemma, one of the staff members supporting Lilly at her Planning Live session, was able to not only share the outcomes and actions with the rest of the team, but also to tell the story of how they had occurred. This ensured that the momentum created at the workshops would continue, and the actions from the planning were implemented the very next week.

Sharing and building a depth of knowledge about the person and how they want to live

It is easy for staff to assume that they know someone really well; however, there are always opportunities to learn more, to see someone with fresh eyes and to hear from others who know and experience the person differently.

Becky's story

Becky, a close support worker of Anne-Marie, worked with Anne-Marie throughout the event along with all the important people in Anne-Marie's life. As a group they went through Anne-Marie's preferences and fully discussed what would help to improve her life. One of the most poignant moments for Becky was hearing what Anne-Marie wanted in her 'perfect day':

> It turned out that one of the things on Anne-Marie's 'perfect day' list was that she'd like to put make-up on every day. That upset me a bit, because I'd worked with her for all these years and it had never occurred to me before Planning Live that she wanted to put make-up on every day. Of course, we did her hair and make-up when we went

out, but without Planning Live and the open environment it created, I don't know if we would have found that out.

For Becky, Planning Live was an absolute turning point, a shift from seeing the week as revolving around the staff rota to one that revolved around what the people being supported needed and wanted.

THE DISADVANTAGES OF PLANNING LIVE

It does not work for everyone

For some people, other ways of support planning definitely work better, and they prefer to plan over a shorter period of time, perhaps with just one or two other people. However, where people do not use words to communicate, this is still a powerful process, as all the people who know and care about the person share their 'best guesses' and the process allows these guesses to be explored and tested. It is easy to assume, for example, that some people will not be able to stay all day; however, there were many examples of how this has been assumed about people but proved not to be the case.

Dora's story

Dora had never shown any interest in any kind of planning meeting. No matter what her team tried, she always opted out by sitting quietly while everyone else spoke. She usually only really spoke up when she had one-to-one time with her staff; therefore, her team was convinced that Dora would not get anything out of Planning Live or want to contribute, and they were worried that they would be doing all the planning for her without really knowing if it was what she really wanted. Juan, the manager, knew that this was an accurate description of how Dora usually responded to meetings, so he was determined to explore the best way to engage her in the process. Dora is a natural homemaker and is never happier than when she is organising things and being hospitable. Juan decided to tap into Dora's skills and actively involve Dora in the overall preparation for the workshops, from making lists for the refreshments, making sandwiches and baking the cakes to posting invitations. As the preparation progressed, Dora showed more interest in what was happening and took more and more ownership and responsibility over her role. She even started to remind the staff team about the schedule.

Despite this preparation, staff were still convinced that at the last minute Dora would say that she would rather not go; however, on the morning of the first day she was ready before anyone else and was waiting at the door ready to go. Throughout the two days staff saw Dora in a new light as she confidently took control of her planning. Dora was open, upfront and clear about what she did and did not want. Staff were delighted to have been proven wrong. Juan, the manager, believes that the preparation was all important, and the overall experience of Planning Live has had a lasting impression as Dora's newfound confidence has continued beyond the workshops. Furthermore, Dora is much more assertive than she used to be.

Logistical challenges

The two-day process can take place over a weekend, but whichever day is chosen, sometimes it is difficult for family members with working and caring commitments. Some Planning Live workshops take place in the person's home, when everyone is involved and there is enough space. Sometimes people use free community rooms, but sometimes there is a cost for a venue to take into account.

Real Life Options used Planning Live to develop all of the support plans as part of the Birmingham Transformation Process. Certitude and Dimensions are using this approach as the main way to build on person-centred information and roll out ISFs. At Bruce Lodge there needed to be a process that was more proportionate to the allocation of two hours a month that individuals had.

One-page profile meetings

Another approach to developing a support plan is the informal meeting approach used at Bruce Lodge. Because individuals living with dementia at Bruce Lodge had only two hours in their individual control, it was very important to make sure the planning process was proportionate to that. Rather than using the full range of person-centred thinking tools found within Planning Live, the 'one-page profile meeting' uses the following person-centred thinking tools (Figure 3.3):

- working and not working from different perspectives

- good days and bad days

- communication chart

- 'If I could, I would'.

From using these person-centred thinking tools in the meeting, there was enough information to complete a one-page profile, clear actions that changed what is not working and how the person wanted to use their individual time.

WHO IS INVOLVED?

The process is usually facilitated by the home manager, with the person themselves, family (if the person has family) and the person's key worker or other staff member who knows them well.

One-page profile meeting

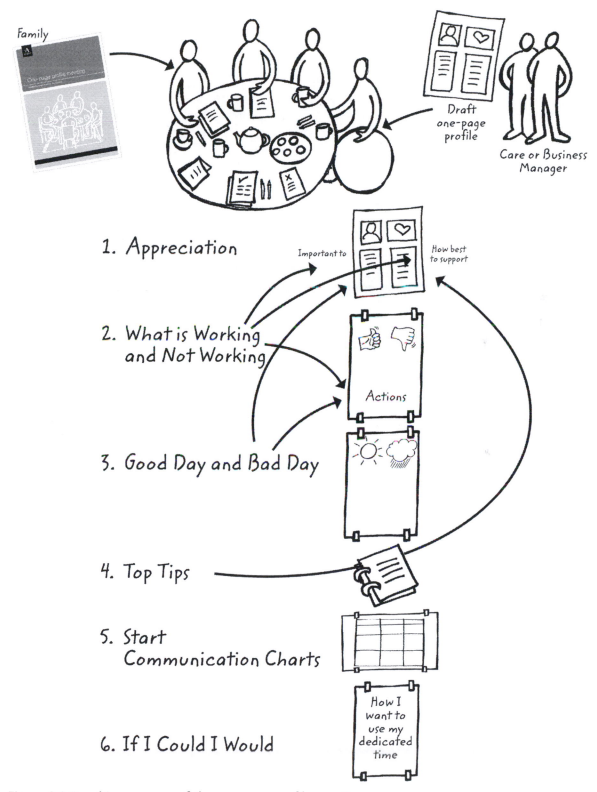

Family

Draft one-page profile

Care or Business Manager

1. Appreciation

Important to

How best to support

2. What is Working and Not Working

Actions

3. Good Day and Bad Day

4. Top Tips

5. Start Communication Charts

How I want to use my dedicated time

6. If I Could I Would

Figure 3.3 Graphic summary of the one-page profile meeting

Mary's story

Mary was born and bred in Gorton (Manchester), a real Mancunian through and through who was described as 'the salt of the earth'. She married Albert (her late husband) and they had four children: Brenda, Maureen, Brian and Karen. Mary was very much a family woman. She raised her children and had various jobs working as a domestic. After her children became adults, Mary remained very close to them, particularly Brenda who visited often. Gill Bailey, who was part of the Leadership Team working on ISFs at Bruce Lodge, describes how this worked with Mary.

Mary was diagnosed with dementia some years ago and went to live in a residential service, Bruce Lodge, which has supported people living with dementia since 2009. As part of a desire within Bruce Lodge to move towards more personalised support, everybody living there was invited to contribute to the development of their one-page profile along with family and staff who knew the person well, and also to think together about how people would want to spend an individual allocation of time each month – two hours to do something they enjoy, at a time and place that suits the person, supported by a member of staff of their choice.

Lisa, the manager of Bruce Lodge, asked if she could meet for an hour with Mary and her daughter Brenda to develop Mary's one-page profile. This was arranged and they met in Mary's room, as this was the place where Mary felt most comfortable. The meeting was held mid-afternoon, as Brenda had said she always found her mother to be at her best at that time of the day.

WHAT HAPPENS?

When family members are able to attend, they are given a booklet that explains what the meeting is for, and questions to help them prepare for it. The meeting is a series of conversations with the person, their family and staff members, for example, talking about what a good day is like, and what a bad day is like now and what it may have been like in the past. This provides information about both, what matters to the person and the support that they need to have more good days and fewer bad days. Furthermore, much is learned in terms of 'If I could, I would' by asking the question, 'If you could do anything in your two hours, what would you do?'

Mary's story (cont.)

The different conversations that Mary and Brenda had were around good days and bad days, and learning what was working and not working. We also focused on Mary's gifts and when the times her well-being was at its best, and we talked about some of the things she might enjoy doing in the future if she could.

What we learned as an 'absolute must' to help promote more good days was to ensure Mary got some chocolate each day. Her daughter, Brenda, said that there's always a supply in a cupboard in her bedroom so that staff could ensure they were offering her chocolate every day. Of course, this information is reflected in her one-page profile to ensure it is present each day and that Mary is consistently supported regardless of the number of staff providing that support.

Mary loves hugs and affection when she's in the mood, and she'll let you know when she's in the mood. She's a very direct woman. She loves to be complimented and enjoys conversation. She'll tell you how she got the possessions she has in her room – the pictures of her family, her CDs, cushions and throws. Having a sing-song is always good. Mary loves to watch the Proms on television, or anything to do with royalty such as changing of the guard.

KEY ELEMENTS OF THE PROCESS

The one-page profile meeting does more than enable people to think about how they want to spend their time. It is a way to gather vital information that can direct how the person is supported on a day-to-day basis; therefore, it is information to learn together, that is, with others who know and care for the person.

Involving family and others who know the person well

Family, friends and staff who know the person well can share important insights and stories to help the person reflect on what matters to them. If the person can no longer tell us directly, then we will be relying on what others can share with us, and if necessary, testing this out. Communication is much more than words, and people living with dementia can tell us a lot about what is important to them through their behaviour, particularly when we are not getting their support right. Some people question whether someone living with dementia would want to, or be able to, sit through a meeting. The experience at Bruce Lodge and other care homes is that it is very important to do everything possible to make the meeting as comfortable and meaningful to the person. As the meeting is intentionally informal, people are usually content to stay, especially when their family is taking part as well. Some organisations give families a preparation booklet to enable them to think and plan what they want to share and feel prepared for the informal meeting.

The manager facilitates the process

The meeting happens through a process of purposeful conversations about good days and bad days, what is working and not working, and what people would like to do in the future, leading to how they would like to use their time. When person-centred planning was first introduced in the UK through Valuing People, many facilitators were trained to use a range of person-centred planning approaches, and lots of person-centred planning meetings took place. At the national annual gathering for person-centred planning facilitators, they would express their frustration at trying to 'hand over' to managers and the difficulty of getting managers to take responsibility for the actions taken as a result of meetings.[2]

When the manager is the person facilitating the meeting, she or he learns firsthand about what is working and not working for the person, is part of generating solutions and has the authority to make sure that those solutions are implemented. A manager's role is to make sure that the best care and support is delivered, and both learning what that means from the person's point of view and hearing what is working and not working about the service at the moment are key for a manager to fulfil this role well. The manager is also responsible for making sure that the individual time goes on the rota.

Being a manager is also an opportunity to coach staff. For example, in Bruce Lodge the leadership team wanted to support people living with dementia to use their individual time within the community, as part of community life, rather than at home. If people really wanted to use their individual time at home, this was supported, but one of the roles of leadership was to have an explicit bias towards, and gently nudge and support, ways that people living with dementia could be connected in their neighbourhood.

---

2   Department of Health (2010) *Personalisation Through Person-Centred Planning.* London: HM Government.

Going beyond life histories

Life stories or life histories are commonly used in person-centred care for people living with dementia. Understanding a person's history is good practice and ensures that we can understand people in the context of their history; however, just because something was important to you in the past does not necessarily mean that it is still important to how you want to live today or in the future; therefore, in support planning we focus on learning what matters to someone *now* and record this in a one-page profile.

Focusing on the future and outcomes

All support planning processes focus on the outcomes that people want to achieve based on assessed needs. Even though this process is proportionate to the amount of time allocated to each individual (two hours), it still needs to identify the outcomes or experiences that people want to have using this time. As suggested earlier, this can be counter-cultural in traditional services supporting people living with dementia.

Lisa's story

Lisa, the manager of Bruce Lodge, also wanted to think with Mary and Brenda about hopes and dreams, something which is often seen as challenging to organisations supporting people living with dementia. This was phrased as 'if I could I would...' and Mary and Brenda talked about this in the context of if they had some time and help, what would Mary like to do? Something that Brenda thought her mother would really enjoy was spending time in the park and also going to cafés. As Mary is in the later stage of her experience of dementia, she has a number of physical needs, so they had to think about what it would take to make this happen for her. Mary loves to watch what is going on when she is outdoors. Due to the amount of physical intervention and bed rest Mary needs, Lisa realised it really was important that staff support Mary to have as many opportunities as possible to go out; therefore, Mary's outcome for her individual time was to go to the park and cafés.

THE ADVANTAGES OF A ONE-PAGE PROFILE MEETING APPROACH

Gathering and acting on information together

The main advantage of a one-page profile meeting is the people connected to the person – family, the manager and staff who know the person well – getting together to share information. This gives an opportunity to share what they love about the person, and for the person to be able to hear this. There are few opportunities in life when we have the chance to be told what people appreciate about us. This is important to well-being. As the meeting process intentionally includes what is working, as well as what is not working, everyone gets to hear the positive information. It is not uncommon for managers to feel that their communication with family members is more likely to be negative than positive, and this process helps redress this a little. Looking at what is not working from different perspectives gives opportunities to see things from each other's point of view, and everyone has the chance to contribute their view to problem-solving and action planning. This is also one of the most time- and cost-effective ways to develop a one-page profile (and begin a communication chart) that has everyone's input and contribution.

Continues building on existing information from a care plan

We know that people who use health and care services are tired of repeating their story and information, again and again, to different people. Before a one-page profile meeting, the manager or key worker reviews all the information in the existing care file to see what is already there that can contribute to the one-page profile. Using this approach, families can feel more confident that they are building on the information they have already shared, and are not simply repeating it.

THE CHALLENGES OF A ONE-PAGE PROFILE MEETING APPROACH

This is the unavoidable consequence to the advantage of people coming together to share and act on information. It can be challenging for the manager to find a date and time that fits with family commitments as well as the availability of the person, the manager and the staff.

We have described different ways to develop support plans (e.g. by basing them on person-centred planning, using approaches to person-centred planning, person-centred thinking tools and Planning Live or one-page profile meetings); however, the support plan is developed with the person, there needs to be a record of both the detailed person-centred information, as well as the outcomes and how this will be achieved.

Recording information in the support plan

Planning Live and one-page profile meetings are ways to gather good person-centred information for support plans. They are ways to think together, explore options and make decisions. The record of this is the support plan. Earlier in this chapter we discussed the seven criteria for developing a good support plan. These criteria are reflected in the support plan recording used by Choice Support, which uses the following headings to record each person's support plan:

- About me and my life

- What is important to me

- What do I want to change or achieve – my outcomes

- How will I stay as healthy, safe and well as I can?

- How will I stay in control of my life?

- How will decisions about my support be made?

SUPPORT PLAN SUMMARY GRID

A support plan summary grid is as follows:

- Outcome (and how this reflected the assessed need, whether it was critical or substantial)

- How I will achieve this outcome

- Contingency plans

- An action plan

- How this will be paid for and how the support will be managed

- Weekly cost

- Annual cost.

Table 3.2 shows an extract from a summary of a support plan.

Table 3.2 *Support plan grid*

Outcomes	Plan	Contingency	Action	How will this be paid for and how will the support be managed?	Weekly cost	Annual cost
Substantial/ critical Part I: keeping myself safe inside and outside of my home.	To put an alarm on the front door to alert staff whenever the door is opened. To support me to learn how to travel safely to my mother's house.	To look into alternative technology to keep me safe.	I will continue to employ my sleep-in supporter. I will ask staff to assist me to contact telecare to install an alarm at my house.	I will share the sleep cost with my two housemates. I will pay with my personal budget, which will be managed by my ISF provider.	7(sleeps) × £** = £*** ÷ 3 = £**.** Cost included in Part N	£**.** × **.*** = £****.** Cost included in Part N

Conclusion

The ISF process starts with allocation, and then support planning is a process to explore and decide how to use the allocation to enable the person to live their life well. In this chapter we have looked at the information that needs to be in a support plan, and how person-centred thinking and planning can contribute, as well as introduced the approaches of Planning Live and one-page profile meetings. The next step in the ISF process is to ensure that this plan is implemented within the budget of the ISF and the other resources available to the individual and their networks. This is what we consider in Chapter 4.

Implementing the Support Plan

Introduction

Reading a good support plan will tell you who the person is, what is important to them, what they want to change about their life and what support they want or need. One of the outputs from Planning Live, for example, is a summary of the person's perfect week (or month), with the amount of flexibility that works for the person. It is very important that the support plan not only describe in detail who the person is and how they want to live, but also what that actually looks like in practice on a daily, weekly and monthly basis. The next step is to see how this week can be delivered within the allocation. The organisations that we looked at either did this in an informal way or several used the process called 'Just Enough Support'.

Just Enough Support

Just Enough Support is a process that turns decision-making about support on its head. Typically, organisations start with the assumption that paid staff are the way to support people. Just Enough Support starts with family, friends, community and assistive technology, and then considers paid staff as an option after that.

The term 'Just Enough Support' means the optimum level of support to enable people to be healthy and safe, and that increases the chances of people connecting with people in their communities. The process aims to ensure that the person's resources are used effectively, and it actively tries to reduce reliance on paid support (while working in ways that enhance relationships and involve people in their community). This can be a win-win situation for:

- the person, who will have a wider variety of connections and relationships

- the organisation, which will be able to target scarce resources most effectively and maximise the use of the budget available to the individual

- the community, which will benefit from the contributions and presence of disabled people.

The process of Just Enough Support involves generating ideas (and asking if they work for the person and provide enough support), testing them in practice and then reviewing them.

Generating ideas

When it comes to generating ideas, many heads are better than one. Ideally, you want to bring together a group where there are people who know the person really well and/or know the area and community where the person lives. Alongside this group, you need one person who knows about assistive technology and someone who can facilitate the process and act as a gentle (or strong) challenge to the group. The person on whom this is focused may want to be part of this, and if they do not, their role is to see if the group's ideas work for them. It is vital to include family members whenever possible and ideally people who do not think in the traditional ways that staff and managers in services often think. (The cliché is 'people who think outside of the box', and however you choose to describe them, it is those people who we mean.) The purpose of the group is to generate ideas that the person will review and decide what they want to try.

The adage 'If you always do what you have always done, you will always get what you have always got' rings especially true here. Doing this process with the existing staff supporting someone, and their manager, is unlikely to come up with as many options as the diverse 'ideas group' described here (but if there is no alternative, start there). Ideally, we need to bring a different group together with a different process to use, to create something different in people's lives.

The following are the four questions the group looks at to generate ideas.

EXACTLY WHAT SUPPORT DOES THE PERSON NEED?

The group accurately describes exactly what support the person needs, how much and how often – not how it is currently provided. For example, instead of stating that the person needs 'waking-night support', we would put that the person needs to be turned four times a night, or needs support if they wake up distressed (and how often this usually is). It can be very useful and illuminating to talk about and understand why we provide some of the support that we do.

WHAT CAN FAMILY, FRIENDS, OTHER PEOPLE OR COMMUNITY INITIATIVES DO THAT COULD HELP?

The best place to start here is with the person-centred thinking tool called the relationship circle, to think together about the people in the person's life. The first place to start is with family. If the person is happy with this, Owen Cooper suggests that we talk to families about their own resources – time, connections, interests, skills and money – and think together about whether any of these resources could be used in ways to support the person. He says, 'Asking families to think about their own resources pays dividends. Worrying about offending people by asking gets in the way'. After family, think about neighbours who live locally and people who share the same interests or go to the same places.

There is a person-centred thinking tool that identifies gifts and contributions, and this helps us to consider whether there are any gifts or resources that could be shared and possibly lead to reciprocal favours. For example, if the person has a car, could they offer lifts to the local church meeting in return for the person offering a bit of support whilst they are there, instead of having paid staff there all the time? The gifts-and-contributions person-centred thinking tool will help you think about gifts or talents that could be useful to other people, and possible opportunities for people to contribute through being good neighbours and taking on responsibility. For example, this could mean taking in parcels for neighbours, holding spare keys or offering their house for neighbourhood watch meetings.

Another person-centred thinking tool that is very helpful is a community map. This is a way to map the places where the person goes already and where there might be opportunities for connections and contributions. The person's relationship map and community map (both person-centred thinking tools) would be used to look at whether family or friends could help. Another area to consider is whether there are local community initiatives that are opportunities to reciprocally share skills, talents and resources. One example is Timebanks. A Timebank is a way to share skills and time across a community, and is based on the principle that everybody has something to offer and its equal. It is a simple equation: an hour of anybody's time is as valuable as an hour of anyone else's time, and that people can offer help to each other in a community through trading hours. If one is not available locally, or not available to everyone, is this an opportunity for the organisation to contribute and be part of making a Timebank available to everyone? Another example is 'Never Watch Alone' in Wigan. This is a way to connect fans with learning disabilities to fellow supporters to attend rugby or football matches.

COULD ASSISTIVE TECHNOLOGY HELP?

When we know exactly what support the person needs, how much and how often, we then need to think about whether assistive technology could help, for example, using bed sensor pads, automatic toilet flushes, motion detectors, automatic links to monitoring stations and call centres. (We explore this further in Chapter 7.)

ARE THERE WAYS WE COULD THINK DIFFERENTLY ABOUT PAID SUPPORT?

There are different models of support to consider. For example, community service volunteers, shared lives, the KeyRing model[1] or other 'life-sharing' possibilities.

Figure 4.1 (page 62) provides a summary of the idea-generation stage and the person-centred thinking tools that can help. In one domain is what is important to the person, and in the other domain is providing enough support. You are obviously looking for ideas that fit into the top-right quadrant. For ideas that fall in the bottom-right quadrant, you could ask what it would take to move them to the top-right quadrant (i.e., is there anything that we could do so that this idea would offer enough support?). Ideas that are on the left side that do not fit with what matters to the person should be discounted. Once you have a list of ideas that look promising, and which the person agrees to explore, you can think more deeply about what the challenges and barriers might be to implementing these ideas, as well as what opportunities they present.

Testing out ideas

Once you have finished the ideas stage, it should be very clear where assistive technology could support the person to achieve what is important to them and the support they need, where friends and family can contribute and where paid staff are still required. After that, the next part of the process is to test out the ideas and then implement the chosen ones. These ideas are tested with the individual (i.e. Do they reflect what is important to you, and do they deliver Just Enough Support?), and one way to test the ideas is to plot them onto a grid like the one in Figure 4.2 (page 63).

---

1   See www.keyring.org.

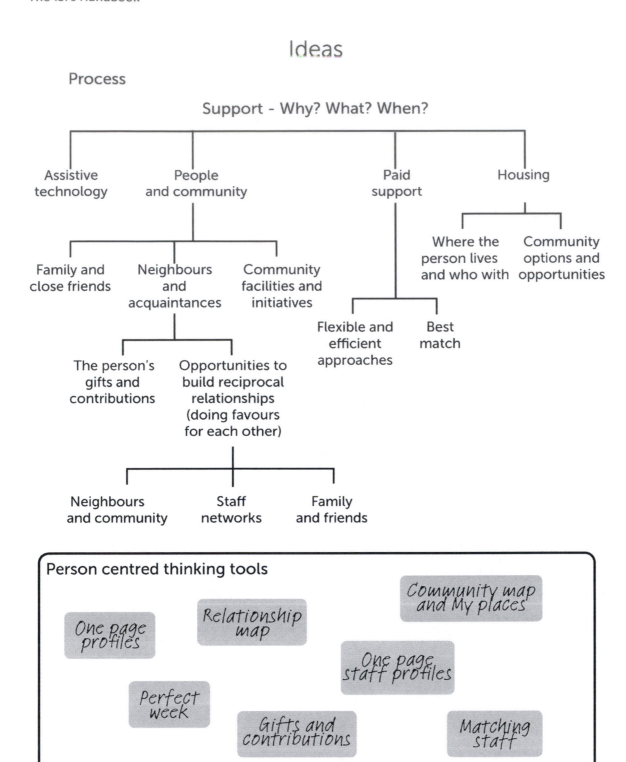

Figure 4.1 Generating ideas in Just Enough Support

Ideas to test

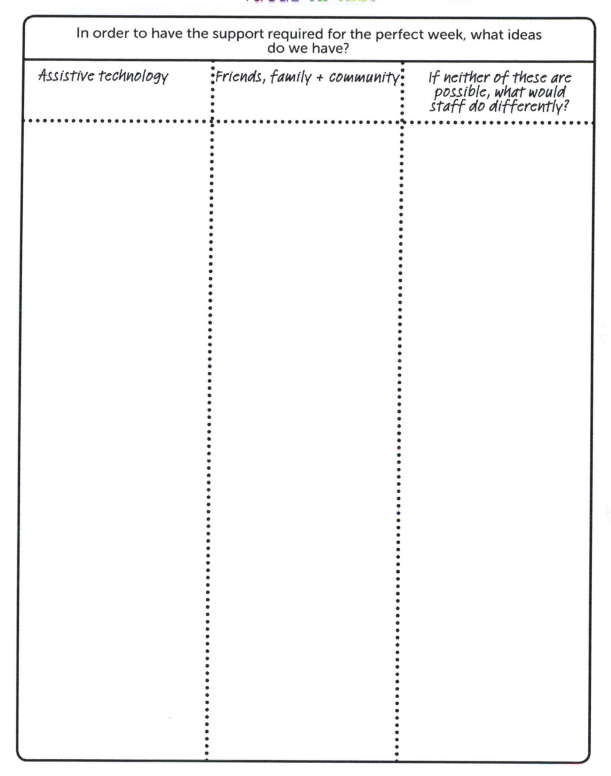

In order to have the support required for the perfect week, what ideas do we have?		
Assistive technology	*Friends, family + community*	*If neither of these are possible, what would staff do differently?*

Figure 4.2 Testing out ideas in Just Enough Support

It is also important to think about what implementing the ideas means, both for the immediate people affected and the wider organisation. What resources might be required? Is any training or support required? Will taking this idea forward require changes to policies and procedures? Will there be any impact on culture or morale as a result of taking this forward?

The next steps are to test out or purchase the assistive technology, negotiate with family and friends whether they are able to do the ideas they have come up with as part of the Just Enough Support process and match staff to the individual regarding how they want to be supported. Chapter 3 introduced Albert and his Planning Live experience, as well as Paul and his support plan. The case study below shows how the Just Enough Support process resulted in a different way of thinking about support for both Albert and Paul.

Albert's story: Just Enough Support

Before Planning Live, Albert's support was focused solely on keeping him healthy and safe. For the Just Enough Support session, Michelle, the team manager, had completed seven support daily records that showed exactly what support he needed. This was applied to the perfect week. For example, due to his skin integrity and susceptibility to pressure areas, Albert needed repositioning every two hours when he was in bed at night. This had been identified as something that was not working for him. As he was being disturbed throughout the night and finding it hard to get back to sleep, this was resulting in his feeling out of sorts and lethargic in the morning. Rather than assuming that two members of staff would be required to facilitate relief for Albert, we used the Just Enough Support process to explore alternatives to paid support. We considered whether assistive technology could help, so an action was recorded to find out. The team was surprised to discover that there was a platform that could be placed under Albert's airflow mattress which could be remotely set to gently reposition him without staff having to physically do this.

Another suggestion for Albert's perfect week was that he try out new things in the community, because Albert had not been going out at all, and staff were not sure what he might like to do. Again, it would have been all too easy to assume that staff would be responsible for finding out what was available; however, we explored whether there were any community initiatives that could help with this. A suggestion was made that the volunteer groups could provide Albert's 'legs in the community', and that this could be a valuable resource for him. Lesley, Albert's key worker, knew that her cousin was taking part in the Duke of Edinburgh awards scheme and asked her if she was interested in taking on this role. Lesley's cousin was pleased to do this and got the added benefit of being able to use the experience towards achieving a Duke of Edinburgh award. Looking at this differently not only resulted in building Albert's resources in the community, but also in his developing a reciprocal relationship beyond his staff team.

Also identified on Albert's perfect week was for him to have storytelling sessions. Although Albert was going to have a much fuller week, his health needs meant that he would still need to rest in bed for certain parts of the day. Staff had come to view these times in quite a task-oriented way, so the aim was for one of these times to be seen as an opportunity for dedicated, quality one-to-one time. This needed to be uninterrupted time that was just for Albert, as he did not want to share this time with others. At the Just Enough Support session it was explored what staff could do differently and the idea of matching the storytelling time to a member of staff who was passionate about books was raised. Cliff, who is a support worker in another service, now visits Albert every Sunday and reads to him for an hour. They are exploring together a whole range of books and poetry as they learn about Albert's literary preferences.

Since Planning Live and Just Enough Support, Albert's week looks radically different. He has new people in his life and shares his love of books with his neighbour as well as his matched staff member. Rather than having his audiobooks delivered to him at home, he enjoys going to choose his own books in the library where he is now a member, after which he stops for a while in the café. His 'legs in the community', Sally, visits once a week and is briefed by Albert and his key worker about what to look out for in the community. He has visited farms in the summer and has been to see shows in the theatre. Due to being repositioned differently, Albert sleeps much better at night, which means that he is more active in the day. This has also resulted in a change in how staffing hours are used.

Paul's story: Just Enough Support

Ruth Gorman, of Imagine, Act and Succeed, describes how she used Just Enough Support to go from Paul's person-centred plan and support plan to deliver the life Paul wanted:

> Paul was very clear about what he wanted to change about his life and how he needed to be included in all conversations and meetings about his future. Paul said that he chose his staff and really liked them all; however, it is very difficult always having someone in your home and not having any time alone. He wanted to be like everyone else. Paul also has a circle and circle facilitator who have been instrumental in supporting the decisions and offering subtle challenges to others if they became a little overprotective. As we knew that assistive technology was going to be a key factor, the local person responsible for this was also asked to contribute. There are some health concerns regarding Paul spending time alone at home and in the community, so it was vital to engage someone from health to participate at the early stages.

Exactly what support does Paul need?

Ruth continues:

> In this Just Enough Support process we accurately describe exactly what support the person needs, how much and how often, not what we currently provide. Paul had already described what would be his perfect day, week and month. We were in a position to balance this against what he currently received. This was done using an hour-by-hour look at his life. He pointed out to us times where he was watching TV and staff didn't need to be around, having a lie-in with staff downstairs in his home, and it became apparent that night-time sleep-ins were questionable. Interestingly, when we unpicked Paul's night-time routine, we were told that Paul was the last person to go to bed at night as he liked to stay up later than the staff, but they would always come down and check that he had locked up. This they admitted was unnecessary, as he had always done a good job, but they thought it was their duty of care. The next time they would speak to Paul or physically see him was when he came down the following morning. One of the justifications for Paul having a sleep-in was that he had epilepsy. The staff member sleeping over would not have known if he had had a seizure, so there were additional requirements. Paul knows his community and neighbours well and is positively seen in his local shop, bookies and when walking his dog. It was very clear that Paul was being over-supported on many occasions.

Could assistive technology help?

Ruth continues:

> Paul visited a 'smart house' (a house with lots of assistive technology in place) in his local area to see what technology was available. An anxiety of the staff was the possibility that Paul could let strangers into his home, as he is such a welcoming person and, in addition, there was the danger of his seizures at night with no staff around. As a result of this, Paul has installed a camera and intercom so that he can see who is at the door before opening it. There is an epilepsy sensor in Paul's bed to alert the on-call duty manager, and this alert also goes to emergency services so that they can be deployed, if needed.

Are there other people or community initiatives that could help?

Ruth continues:

> For Paul, his only family is his nephew who lives in New Zealand. Paul keeps in touch with him through his computer; he uses Skype and e-mail to let his nephew know the changes in his life. Paul always says that his mother would be very proud if she could see him now.
>
> One relationship that was identified by Paul and his team as being crucial is that with his dog, Poppy. The staff noted that they were worried about Paul getting distracted when out in the community on his own, as this sometimes happens when he has support. 'What if he walks into the road?' was asked. This created a significant conversation, and as the discussion unfolded it seemed that Paul never did this when he had Poppy with him, as he was worried about her getting run over. Could Poppy become the companion when Paul is out and about, and act as a fantastic natural support?
>
> Paul had tried many times over the years to build a relationship with his neighbour, and it could be a possibility that because he always had a staff member with him, that in itself had become the barrier. The neighbour's wife died and Paul worried that this elderly neighbour was not going out as much as he had. Paul started to knock at the door when he was going to the local shops to enquire if the neighbour needed anything. For a long time, the neighbour refused. It was only during one of these conversations that Paul mentioned also going to the betting shop to place a bet that the commonality became apparent. They discovered that this was the thing that they had in common and soon broke down barriers. Paul regularly shops and places bets now for both of them, and the neighbour is someone Paul can go to if he needs assistance during the day or night. This is a very reciprocal relationship that is borne out of a mutual interest and respect.
>
> Paul has a love of gardening and has started his own micro-enterprise. He produced a business plan with some support from his team and applied for a small setup grant from his provider. The fund that he applied for was the community innovation fund that had been set up to support such initiatives. Paul now grows salad, vegetables and flowers, and he undertakes gardening for others. He has gone to other neighbours in his street to give some of his produce away (he sells the rest) and feels that he is really contributing. He would describe himself as a fair-weather gardener, though, as he gardens spring through to autumn only. Paul has been thinking through the idea of setting up a home-watch scheme and will continue to consider that.

Are there ways we could think differently about paid support?

Ruth continues:

> From Paul's perspective, the ideas that we had started to implement and all the additional new ones were supportive. Previously, Paul had support with him 24 hours a day and that needed to change; everyone recognised and acknowledged this. Paul did understand this would have implications on his staff team. Staff would have to become much more flexible. They would no longer be working in large blocks of time, as Paul was clear about where and when he wanted his support. It was, at times, difficult for the staff, as although they felt that this was great for Paul, they were being replaced by a dog, a neighbour and technology. Naturally, there was a sense of loss as Paul had chosen them to work with him. This was not a barrier that stopped the implementation but instead a factor to consider. The provider had to accommodate the change in hours, rotas and the flexibility around this to enable it to happen.
>
> In addition, Poppy has become the natural support when out and about, and as any dog lover knows, you always get to chat to others who also have dogs. This has

enhanced Paul's community presence. He and the people around him were very clear about what was to happen next, and there was a nervous excitement for everyone.

The provider had to think very carefully about staff morale, and currently they are revising their policy regarding friendships and relationships. It is important that the whole process be transparent and engage the right people early in the process to ensure acceptance and participation.

Paul now has a new rota. He completes this on a four-weekly basis with the team leader. He no longer has 24-hour support but instead support that is tailored to meet his needs. The implementation issues around this are picked up through job consultation and team meetings. Paul lets the team leader know his views beforehand and is included for some of the job consultation and all of the team meetings.

One of the keys in making this approach work was ensuring that all the assistive technology needed was in place and all possible eventualities covered. We cannot plan for everything, and one of the surprising things that happened early was that Paul's electrics fused. Paul put Poppy on her lead and walked round to another tenancy where we support people and asked for their assistance. Paul did not feel he needed to phone the on call duty manager as he had it under control, which shows his capability for using his initiative. One of the obvious realities in this process is that if we demonstrate to people that we believe in their capacity, the person shines.

Although the staff were initially worried about how Paul would cope, their fears have been alleviated and the staff team has been a shining example of people who truly understand their role and purpose in a person's life. They have since said that they did worry about how this would affect them and their work. We took the time to really engage with them at every point, did not dismiss their fears, either for Paul or themselves, and it has paid dividends.

The 'win' for Paul is pretty obvious: he was listened to, we acted upon it and he is more independent and confident as a result. He chooses when to have his support and does not feel like he has someone looking over his shoulder 24 hours a day. His relationship with his neighbour has blossomed as a result, he is seen as a helpful member of his local community and he has his loyal companion, Poppy. I know that some people will look at this situation and say, 'What happens when Poppy dies?' We will cross that bridge when we get to it. Right now life is as good as it's ever been for Paul and he is in control.

From a provider perspective, the 'win' is that we are truly providing a service that is driven by the person. The staff understand their role in Paul's life and are flexible as a result. Paul's story inspires others in the organisation to take more control of their lives. Paul's service was undoubtedly an expensive one when it was originally set up, and that was right for him at that time after spending over 50 years in a hospital; however, we have been able to say to the local authority that the service he receives is of a much higher quality and the cost of his support has now halved.

The local authority sees this as a 'win' because the service is of high quality, Paul is very happy, the risks have been managed in a person-centred way and they now have half of the cost of Paul's package, which can be put to good use to support another person.

Choosing staff

Once the team has finished exploring opportunities to use assistive technology, friends, family and community, the next step is for the person to choose the staff they want to support them in their perfect week. This could either be choosing from the existing staff team or recruiting new staff. Michelle matched staff to Albert's interests, for example, a staff member who loved books and reading to Albert.

Below are two other examples of how individuals can choose their own staff to support them to deliver their perfect week.

Anne-Marie's story: Choosing staff

A team of 16 people supported both Anne-Marie and the other five people with whom she lived. These people were not whole-time equivalents, but it did mean that 16 different people were coming and supporting Anne-Marie and her colleagues. In order to work out with Anne-Marie who she wanted to support her, the first thing that Carolynn (the manager) did was identify who Anne-Marie wanted in her team, and to do this they used the relationship map. Carolynn sat down with Anne-Marie with three concentric circles in front of them with Anne-Marie's name in the middle circle.

The first question Carolynn asked was, 'Who are the people who feel really good when they're coming on shift that you look forward to seeing or you have the most fun with?' Anne-Marie identified four staff members and told Carolynn their names.

The next question Carolynn asked was, 'Who are the staff members you're pleased to see – and it's fine when they're on shift – that are not quite as special as these four people here? Who are the other people you're really happy to support you?' Anne-Marie chose everybody else in the staff team, except one person.

Then Carolynn asked, 'Is there anybody you would prefer not to support you?' Anne-Marie identified the remaining member of staff.

The next task for Carolynn and Anne-Marie was to look at how Anne-Marie wanted to spend her perfect week, that is, how close they could get for a good match between what Anne-Marie wanted to do and the hobbies and interests of the four staff members she had chosen.

The leadership team that was supporting this to happen 'acted like detectives' as they looked at all the activities and interests that clearly made Anne-Marie's perfect week, and then looked at the one-page profiles of the four staff that Anne-Marie had selected to see how far it was possible to get a good match. Some of that worked really well and fairly easily.

One thing Anne-Marie wanted to do was to learn how to bake. (On one staff member's one-page profile was the fact that she loved cooking, so this was an easy match.) Something else that Anne-Marie wanted to do was to set up a social enterprise of dog walking. One of the people she had chosen to be in her team loved dogs and walked his own dogs (so again, an easy match). Of course, all of the matches were not that simple. But Carolynn and the team went as far as they could to get the best match between what Anne-Marie wanted to do during her week and the ideal person to support her to do it based on shared interests from the four people she had chosen.

Carolynn's task was to put that information into a personalised rota to get the consistency of who Anne-Marie wanted to support her, and doing which task on which day of the week. As you can imagine, that was a reasonably complex way of doing a rota.

Ken's story: Choosing staff

The second approach is the one used at Bruce Lodge. Through the informal meeting to develop the one-page profile and identify how the person wanted to spend their two hours, what Lisa (the manager) had gathered were the specific interests the person would like to do in their two hours, and whether they wanted to use it in half-hour blocks each week, an hour every other month or in a block of two hours together.

Bruce Lodge staff did not only have a one-page profile; they had a second sheet called 'If I could, I would'. So Lisa had information at her fingertips of what was important to each member of staff (their hobbies, interests and passions) and also what else they would like to do if they had the opportunity.

These were not things like going to Australia or on a hot air balloon ride. We specifically asked staff to think about local things that they would really like to become involved in or try that could be done in about two hours.

Ken is an ex-professional footballer with Stockport County, a fun-loving man with dementia who, for the past three years, has lived at Bruce Lodge. Ken's family sat down with him and some of the team members who knew him best to discuss what they could do to help him, as he appeared to have lost his zest for life and fun. They had several conversations together and developed a one-page profile with Ken. What emerged as really important to Ken were things such as sharing his Stockport County memorabilia and old photos, watching football on TV and having people around him with which to enjoy banter. Ken will always seek people out and be 'amongst it', as he says. Lisa looked for someone to match with Ken who was also interested in football, who Ken really got on with, and she chose Sarah. Sarah had never been to a football match and had always wanted to go: she had listed 'go to a football match' on the 'If I could I would' section of her one-page profile. This enabled Ken to be the expert and introduce his passion to Sarah, an opportunity for someone living with dementia to be and feel useful, have a purpose and make a contribution. Ken said, 'Going to the football again was belting – I felt like I was out there on the pitch again' and 'It's smashing going with Sarah'.

Recruiting new staff

Implementation can also begin by recruiting staff. The support plan can be used as the basis for recruiting staff to work with the individual. Sometimes the individual is 'recruiting' staff from within the existing staff pool, as Anne-Marie's story describes, to be part of his or her individual team. At other times, the individual will be recruiting new staff to the provider specifically to work with the individual as part of their team.

Providers need to use the support plan to work with the individual to develop:

- a person specification
- a job description
- a local recruitment and selection process
- a contract for individual staff
- a contract with the organisation.

Georgia's story: Recruiting staff

One of the managers, Georgia, describes the process that they use to recruit staff to individuals who have an ISF:

> Not unlike many providers, we have struggled to recruit staff on behalf of the people we support in a way that feels really inclusive. We have experimented with many different initiatives, some successful and others good attempts. What we have learned is that for some people, being meaningfully involved in choosing staff is a real challenge.
>
> We knew that a lot of well-intentioned best-guessing was happening around matching staff skills to people using our services. We decided to have a go at figuring out how we could do this better, particularly for those people who choose not to sit on an interview panel. We needed to learn how we could go from the information in a support plan to develop a person specification, a job description and to use this to meaningfully select staff. This is the process that is used with people who have a personal budget used as an ISF.

The person develops their recruitment file from their support plan or person-centred plan. The contents of this file are as follows:

- my person specification

- my one-page profile

- who is in my life (relationship circle)

- what the characteristics are of the people I'd like to work with me

- my perfect week.

When a new member of staff is needed, the position is advertised locally by word of mouth, in the newspaper, in shop windows, in job centres and so forth. Submitted applications are short listed based on the information contained in the person specification and the 'What are the characteristics of the people I'd like to work with me?' sections.

Interviewing is a two-step process. New staff are recruited to the organisation first, to ensure that they have the values and talents required to fit the organisation. Only people who meet these requirements are available to be selected by the individual as part of their own staff team. The two steps are as follows:

- Step one is the formal interview (recruiting to the organisation).

   The person or people wanting staff take part only if it makes sense to them; otherwise, team leaders along with family members or support staff take care of this stage. If the person being interviewed meets our organisational values and standards, they are sent on to phase two of the interview. It is usually the case that three or four candidates get this far.

- Step two is the informal interview (recruiting to the individual).

   Each person or small group of people sharing support determine the best environment for this to take place. It is usually somewhere familiar and comfortable for the person looking for new staff. The two men who live at 'The Way' chose to use a local pub to check out their prospective staff. People closest to the individual(s) are invited to help with this stage of the process, as they most likely would have been involved in the development of the recruitment file and are therefore aware of the person's wishes and what is important to them. An informal series of conversations take place, photos are taken of candidates, and then the person chooses which of the candidates they want to join their team.

Although this process seems pretty simple, it involved a real shift in our thinking. We needed to balance our legal responsibilities as employers with the belief that recruitment should be led by those requiring support. In the past we would have chosen the best candidate based on a generic process and what we thought would be the best match. This new process ensures that the people we support are consulted and listened to from the outset and have the final say.

Jennie's story: Using the support plan to inform recruitment

Independent Options and Jennie's family and circle needed to recruit staff to support Jennie. They were able to use the information directly from Jennie's support plan to develop the person specification and job description. Suzie, Jennie's mother, describes how this happened:

To keep Jennie at the centre of selecting staff meant that we needed to start with the person specification and job description, and make sure that this was specific to Jennie. We used the person-centred thinking tool 'Matching' to think about the kind of person who would be the best match for Jennie. Her support plan described the characteristics that someone who worked with Jennie would need. This meant thinking about the support Jennie needed, the skills that someone would need, what kind of person they would need to be (personality characteristics) and what kind of interests they should share with Jennie. There was no point in choosing someone who didn't like horses because they wouldn't want to take her riding, and the same went for Jennie's other interests such as swimming and going for walks. This gave us the person specification.

Person Specification for Jennie's Support
Senior Support Worker

Matching staff

Personality Characteristics Needed	Support Needed	Skills Needed for the post (Essential requirements)	Shared Interest (Desirable requirements)
• Punctual • Adaptable • Calm • Patient • Good Listener • Trustworthy • 'Firm but Fair' approach • Confident • Leadership skills • Organisational skills **All assessed using the application form, activity interview and panel interview**	• To support Jennie in her weekly activity, going with her to all activities and supporting her in them • To communicate with Jennie using visual supports and her communication charts • To support Jennie in her friendships and relationships • Work with Jennie's family and Trust Circle to share and record information and learning • Support Jennie in her daily routines • Support Jennie with her personal care needs • Helping Jennie to maintain a healthy lifestyle • Support Jennie using the support plan and person-centred plan • To support Jennie by giving positive encouragement as well as setting firm boundaries when necessary • To support Jennie to manage her own home • To support Jennie to be safe within the home and outside **Not assessed**	• Good communication skills, using visual supports to do this where appropriate • Good interpersonal skills and ability to relate well to others • Able to deliver flexible, sensitive support working to Jennie-centred plan, in a consistent way • Able to write accurate reports • Able to use a computer including Microsoft Office • Able to assist in the planning and budgeting of menus and meals • Able to work in a 'Firm but Fair' approach • Personal commitment to valuing and respecting people's rights, choices and dignity • Able to carry out domestic tasks and manage finances • Able to satisfy an Enhanced CRB disclosure • Able to work as part of a team • Able to use own initiative • Personal flexibility and ability to work days, evenings, waking nights, sleep in duties, weekends and bank holidays on a rota system • Able to motivate self and others • Minimum of 2 years' experience working with people with learning disabilities and/or autism • Car driver with clean driving licence **Assessed using application form, group interview, activity interview and panel interview**	• Horse riding • Walking • Going to the gym • Cinema • Art activities • Bowling • Using a computer, for example using YouTube • Music (80s pop music) • Trampolining • Going to places of interest, for example, Chester Zoo **Assessed using the application form and activity interview** **Other Desirable Requirements** • Previous experience of supporting people with Autism • Knowledge of the Stockport area • NVQ level 3 in Health and Social Care • Experience of supervising staff • Experience of maintaining a staff rota • Ability to support individuals with their finances **Assessed using application form and panel interview**

Figure 4.3 Person specification for Jennie's support

Conclusion

So far in this book we have looked at allocation, ways to develop support plans and how to implement support plans through Just Enough Support, which means making sure people look at a range of ways to provide the support that someone needs, thinking about relationships, assistive technology and community. The next step is to record what has been agreed, learn from implementation and then review progress. Chapter 5 looks at how to do this through person-centred reviews.

Chapter 5

Review

Introduction

The process for developing Individual Service Funds (ISFs) starts with allocation and then progresses to planning, agreement, implementation and finally review. The person-centred review is not the end of the process; instead, it is the point where the cycle starts again. The person-centred review is a way to look at what is working and not working in relation to achieving outcomes, support, finances and any other areas of the person's life. From this information we can think about the following:

- What needs to change to maintain what is working and change what is not working?

- Does anything need to change about the allocation?

- What needs to change or be updated in the support plan, and what are the person's outcomes for the following year?

- What would therefore need to be changed or updated in the person's 'perfect week'?

- How can we deliver these changes with the person using 'Just Enough Support'?

- How can we implement this, and who needs to do what?

The person-centred review is where the organisation accounts to the person about their allocation and how it is being spent. The majority of the organisations we learned with were either already using or introducing the person-centred review process as their way to reflect on learning and review progress. In this chapter we examine the review process and explore it in practice for David, who has mental health issues, Anne-Marie and Jean, who lives at Bruce Lodge.

Person-centred reviews

With people who have had an ISF for a while, a person-centred review is a way to check whether it is really leading to greater choice and control for the person. For some people, it is a way to kick-start greater person-centred changes in the person's life. For David, who is supported by Mercy Cole and her team from Certitude, a person-centred review has been instrumental in helping him build a new life for himself.

David's story: Person-centred review

Mercy explains how David has been helped:

> When David came to live with us in 2010 we could see he wasn't completely happy, so we invited his social worker and other people who were important and close to him for a person-centred review. We found out that most of all David likes to be busy and occupied. He was bored by the repetitive nature of his days and wanted to spend less time at a day centre where he was going five times a week. He also didn't want to be spending every weekend back with his parents; he wanted to be out doing things with people his own age.

> We had to think creatively and carefully to support him to do more of what he wanted within the budget he was allocated. He now has a job at the café in Ealing Hospital where he goes once a week, and we hooked him up with 'Out and About' which is a Certitude project which brings people together to go to the places they want such as theatre trips, pubs, football matches or just a coffee. At weekends, David now usually meets up with friends or goes to watch Queens Park Rangers football matches.
>
> The person-centred review was the start of a transformation for David which we've all watched with interest. David is in his late thirties, but before it was like he was living the life *others* wanted for him. Now he is living his own life. He's getting to know himself and is much more able to let us know what he wants. He is much more expressive and tells us what he wants. Nothing is fixed and we can change around him.

A person-centred review typically takes place either annually or every six months. It is an opportunity to look at how the person is spending their money (or allocation of hours), how we are doing in achieving the original outcomes that were identified through support planning and what is working and not working from the person's and staff's perspectives, and possibly the perspectives of the social worker and family. A person-centred review is a meeting that takes about 90 minutes. It starts with the individual – and whoever is supporting them to do the review – looking at their relationship circle and identifying who they want to attend their review, and when and where they want the review to take place. The person who is facilitating the review takes time to think about what it will take for the individual to feel truly at the centre of their person-centred review and how they want to contribute to the review. The friends, family and staff who the person wants to invite to the review are invited ideally by the person themselves, or if not, by staff on the person's behalf.

The person-centred review is a structured, facilitated process that enables people to contribute what they appreciate about the person since they were last together, add any information about what is important to the person that would have taken place over the previous six months and anything new people have learned about how best to support the person. They think together with the person about what they might want to do in the future, what is working and not working from different perspectives and any questions to look at together.

The facilitator then works with the group to look at celebrating what is working well, and also asking questions regarding what will it take to keep this happening. They look at what is not working, where the person wants to be in a year's time that would be different from what is not working and what actions we need to take to get them there. The facilitator also checks whether the way the person is using their allocation is still the way they want to use it, and what might need to change if that is not the case. Sometimes this may require a re-assessment or a review of the allocation. The person-centred review therefore is a way to update the support plan, and this has a knock-on effect on the perfect week and implementation overall.

The case study below demonstrates what the person-centred review process looked like for Anne-Marie and then for Jean.

Anne-Marie's story: Person-centred review

The person-centred review process begins, like most things, with good preparation. For Anne-Marie this meant thinking about when and where she wanted to have the review and who she wanted to invite. It was also a good time for Anne-Marie to start to look at her outcomes and to think about what she wanted to share in the review, and how she wanted to do this.

Anne-Marie prepared by talking this through with her support worker, and Carolynn talked her through the preparation booklet and the headings informally over a cup of tea. Carolynn supported her to invite her father and the staff who she wanted to attend. She wanted to have the meeting on a Wednesday afternoon – she goes to a class in the morning, and wanted to have it after that. In a person-centred review, the person shares their own perspective and then everyone adds their information (including family and friends). So, rather than sitting formally around a table, information is shared and built together. Sometimes flipchart paper is pinned on the walls in the room and everyone is given a pen so that they can write their thoughts on each subject in a more relaxed way.

Information is recorded around the following questions:

- What were Anne-Marie's outcomes for a year?

- What worked and did not work for each of them?

- What is working and not working generally for Anne-Marie, and from others' perspectives?

- What is important to Anne-Marie now – is there anything that we need to change in her one-page profile and support plan?

- What is important to Anne-Marie for the future, and what are her new outcomes for the next year?

- How has Anne-Marie spent her personal budget?

- What questions do we need to answer?

This process is also used with 'what else we need to learn' by looking at the 'questions to answer' and then thinking about any person-centred thinking tools that could help address those questions. The record and information from the person-centred review is written up or photographed and produced in whatever way is required. On the day that the review was organised, Anne-Marie did not feel like spending time with people and did not want the review to take place in the way that had been planned. Carolynn discussed this with her, and in the end, Anne-Marie decided that she wanted to have a chat at the local café with just one person instead. Anne-Marie talked about each of her outcomes and what was working and not working about each one. This feedback was then built into actions for the team to work on with Carolynn. The section of the review on how Anne-Marie was spending her money, and getting the perspective of her family, happened later through separate conversations rather than a meeting. Anne-Marie wanted to think about what she wanted to achieve over the next year at a later date. It was very important that we reviewed the outcomes with Anne-Marie, accounted to her about her money and sought the perspectives of her family and others. It was also crucial that although Anne-Marie had prepared for her meeting, on the day itself we completely respected her decision to achieve this in a different way.

Below are some examples of what we learned with Anne-Marie and what has changed in her life.

Some outcomes had been successful

One of Anne-Marie's outcomes was to walk dogs as a job. She was now doing this, walking a dog called Gem, and she was getting paid. She found that there were aspects of walking a dog that she did not like but loved the dog walking overall and enjoyed having money, which she was saving.

Another very successful outcome was spending more time with her father. Anne-Marie now sees her father once a fortnight, and in between visits she phones him and is supported to write to him or send him a card. Her father also visits her at home and her relationship with him is much closer, and Anne-Marie is really pleased about this.

Anne-Marie also wanted to work in a tea room or a café. The team supported her to experience this as a volunteer first, so that Anne-Marie could decide whether she wanted to keep doing this as a volunteer or to explore this as a paid job. Anne-Marie is a volunteer at the church coffee morning every Sunday. She loves the social side of this and has made new friends who now stop for a chat if they bump into each other in the village. Anne-Marie has been asked to help at the church fête as a direct result of her work at the coffee morning. She is now part of the church community and wants to continue this, even if eventually she wants to get a paid job as well.

Some outcomes had not been completely successful

Anne-Marie wanted to be in touch with her sister. The staff supported her to send cards and to phone. For the first time in six years, Anne-Marie got both a Christmas card and a birthday card from her sister, and she was delighted. Her original outcome was to see or speak to her sister, and although this has not happened yet, a first step has been made.

Some outcomes changed as Anne-Marie explored them over six months

One of Anne-Marie's outcomes was to go out more for meals and to the theatre. Anne-Marie goes out each week about three times for meals, tea or coffee. Over six months, staff could not find anything at the theatre that Anne-Marie wanted to see. She has been going to the cinema a couple of times a month. As part of the review process, she said that she now wanted to go to a pub to see live music and go to a musical.

Anne-Marie wanted to extend some of her outcomes

Another of Anne-Marie's outcomes was to look good and wear make-up. If you met Anne-Marie, you would see that she wears make-up most of the time and has her nails painted each week. Anne-Marie has what she calls 'pamper sessions' every week and enjoyed a 'pamper evening' organised by the local church. Now that wearing make-up and having her nails painted is part of her daily and weekly routine, she wants to extend that to having her hair dyed every six weeks.

Some outcomes Anne-Marie no longer wants to achieve in the same way

Anne-Marie wanted to learn how to bake and wanted to bake every week. She bakes cakes, biscuits and other items every couple of weeks. (Early on, she made it clear that once every two weeks was enough, despite its being originally planned for every week.) In her review conversation she said that she did not want to bake anymore; instead, she wants to cook, starting with a curry dish.

Carolynn then went back to the 'perfect week' with Anne-Marie to make the changes that she wanted. Anne-Marie's life now looks more like that of other women of a similar age who live in the same area. She volunteers at her local church, dances, goes to the cinema and out for meals, tea and coffee, and sees her father.

Anne-Marie earns a bit of money through her dog walking and is saving for a holiday. The big difference is that she lives with people who have a disability. She is much more in control of her service, she chooses her staff, says what she wants to do and when, and the staff are accountable to Anne-Marie in making the changes to her life that she wants to make. Anne-Marie's relationship with her father and his partner has improved and they now have more regular, positive contact. She also enjoys seeing her partner, Terry, more regularly at her request. (They have been out for several meals together, and she also likes preparing meals for him at home.)

Through being part of her local community, Anne-Marie has developed friendships with other people too. She visits them at their homes, invites them to visit her or they meet up for coffee at various local cafés. Only one of the groups that Anne-Marie attends is specifically for people with learning difficulties and is run by an advocacy group. She has chosen to keep attending this group, rather than try something else, and she has made a good friend there who she sees regularly.

Anne-Marie takes the central role in planning what she does and has become very good at using photos to decide where to go, for example, when she is deciding which supermarket in which location she wants to shop. She has developed skills in money management, so she understands what she can and cannot afford to do. She has also become more confident and less anxious, including being more assertive in making decisions.

Jean's story: Person-centred review

Gill Bailey, part of the leadership team at Bruce Lodge, describes Jean's person-centred review:

> Jean's home is at Bruce Lodge with other people who live with dementia. Jean's one-page profile meeting took place in February, and in July, we met again with Jean and her family to have a person-centred review. Jean wanted to use her individual time to go to church, and she was matched with Olivia, who shared the same faith. As she had two hours a month, this meant that she could attend Mass once a month. We looked at some of the things that were working and not working for Jean, and we developed ways of addressing any problems. Below is a description of the things that weren't working and what we did to correct them.

Going to church
Gill continues:

> We learned at Jean's person-centred review that she wasn't going to Mass and church events every week. She had always belonged to St Vincent de Paul, so we decided that Olivia would speak with the chair of the St Vincent de Paul Society at St Joseph's to explore the possibility of one of the members of the Society getting to know Jean. We hoped that the Society member would support Jean to go to meetings with a view to making more friends who would be able to call for her each Sunday morning so she could go to Mass.

Poetry
Gill continues:

> Jean loves poetry and we learned at the review that she wasn't having the opportunity to listen to her poetry, and staff weren't able to find the time to sit and read poetry to her. The team thought about this and decided that Sue, a care staff member and Jean would go to the local library and bookstores to try to find some audiobooks by Jean's favourite poets to which she could listen.

Moving around
Gill continues:

> We also learned, because Jean's niece told us, that Jean was struggling more and more to open the doors and get around the building with a walking frame that seemed to be very cumbersome. We had some discussion around this, and decided that Kerri, the deputy manager, would make a referral for an occupational therapy assessment to

consider other walking aids that might be less cumbersome than Jean's walking frame so that she could get about much more freely.

After the person-centred review, Lisa updated Jean's one-page profile from the new learning we gained during the meeting and made sure that it was shared with all staff.

In summary, person-centred reviews at Bruce Lodge resulted in:

- an updated one-page profile with information and other changes that the person wants

- a new understanding about what's working and not working from different perspectives

- actions to change what's not working and to build on what is working

- a new or updated outcome for the person's individual time.

Person-centred reviews are a space to stop and reflect. They are an opportunity to look together at what is working and not working for the person, and for people providing support, as well as family and friends. The person-centred review is one of the ways that the organisation is accountable to the person. It reveals both, how the allocation is being used and progress on outcomes. It is where the process cycles back into reviewing the allocation, if needed, and updating the support plan with what has been tried and learned as well as what the person wants to do next.

Conclusion

In Section 1 we have outlined the process of allocating an ISF for individuals and how to use this as the starting point for developing and implementing a support plan based on what is important to the individual. In Section 2 we move beyond the individual process to think about the organisational changes that have been made by the organisations to support the successful delivery of ISFs across the organisation.

Key Issues and Learning in Implementation

Chapter 6

Managing the Change

Introduction

Organisational change is a complicated and difficult process, with research estimating that 70 per cent of change programmes do not succeed in practice. Change in health and social care organisations has its own unique dimensions due to the nature of the work that the organisations undertake and the strong value base that underpins their work. Being committed to the principles of personalisation requires that organisations have the interests of the individuals using their services and their families at their centre of these changes. They also need to respond to the expectations of their commissioners and to maintain a stable and committed workforce. In this chapter we reflect on the approaches taken by the organisations to generate and sustain momentum for the changes connected with ISFs.

Organisations

BOROUGH CARE LTD

A Borough Care Ltd leadership team was created to oversee the project with the key representatives from three partners who would be responsible for facilitating and directly implementing the process (Box 6.1). Facilitated by Helen Sanderson Associates (HSA), the purpose of this team was to implement the principles of ISFs in a way that did not cost the commissioners or the provider more money (i.e. within existing resources). The only additional cost was the input from HSA, which was funded by the commissioner. The leadership team included two representatives from the Stockport Council who were primarily present to gather learning for wider roll-out of ISFs. These representatives were the workforce lead (to learn what would need to change in the way staff were supported to better implement personalisation and ISFs in care homes), and the contracts and quality lead (to learn about what adjustments may be needed in their contract interactions with providers). There was also a member from Stockport Council's communication team, whose role was to support the sharing of information across Stockport Council, and with other stakeholders.

Box 6.1 Borough Care Ltd leadership team

Borough Care Ltd: Chief executive, deputy chief executive and home manager.

Stockport: Integrated commissioner, head of service, workforce lead, contracts and quality lead, and communications officer.

HSA: Consultant and trainer, Helen Sanderson, who facilitated the project and leadership team meetings, and Gill Bailey, who provided direct support to Bruce Lodge.

The group met for a full day, monthly, for the first six months and then for half a day each month after that. Before beginning the work to introduce ISFs, Bruce Lodge developed a baseline of current practice within the home. This baseline included dementia care mapping with the support of an external mapper, direct observations of the resident's quality of life and an assessment by the home manager of the current practices and processes in the home (Progress for Providers for Managers). In the first meeting, the group developed a one-page strategy. This involved identifying what success looked like for each stakeholder in this process (people, staff, Borough Care Ltd and Stockport Council), how this success would be delivered and how they would measure how they were doing. The six steps in developing ISFs were used as the overall framework for the changes, and a dashboard was developed that was updated and shared at each meeting to report on progress.

CERTITUDE

The first stage of getting the ISF project underway was to seek approval to proceed from the Certitude board. Away days were organised to provide information on ISFs and give the trustees an opportunity to raise questions and concerns. A project lead was identified with a background in person-centred working and who had previously been responsible for developing person-centred support within Certitude. A project board was set up, with work streams to progress with the cross-cutting issues of communication, human resources, and finance and contracting, as well as operational leads to take forward the changes within the different service areas. The ISF project board was accountable to the Certitude board through regular reports by directors. Over time, the ISF project board has begun to oversee other projects within the organisation such as 'community connecting' and 'creative communication'. Local authorities were not asked to be members of the project board, but attempts were made to engage them in the change process. This led to one commissioner becoming actively engaged, but (as expected) the changes within and pressures on other authorities meant that it was not initially possible to secure their interest.

CHOICE SUPPORT

The enormity of the challenge was recognised from the outset and was likened to an 'internal re-provision' programme on the scale of previous closures of long-stay NHS facilities. An experienced director who had overseen major change projects in the past was seconded to lead the programme. He was accountable to a steering group drawn from the local authority and family member representatives, and worked with a group of local managers to plan and coordinate the required actions. There was also a funding panel of commissioners and care managers to approve the funding process and packages. A three-year project plan was drawn up and submitted to the commissioners, and they were then willing for Choice Support to take the lead with regular reporting on progress. The ADKAR change management model was used as a framework to plan the changes (Box 6.2).[1]

---

1   See also www.change-management.com/tutorial-adkar-overview-mod1.htm, accessed 1 July 2014.

> # Box 6.2 ADKAR model of change
>
> Prosci's[2] ADKAR model is an individual change management model. It outlines the five building blocks of successful change, whether that change occurs at home, in the community or at work. ADKAR is an acronym based on the five building blocks:
>
> - **A**wareness of the need for change
>
> - **D**esire to participate and support the change
>
> - **K**nowledge on how to change
>
> - **A**bility to implement required skills and behaviours
>
> - **R**einforcement to sustain the change.

The project board recognised the importance of involving front-line managers and staff in the change process, and that this needed to be more than just informing them of what was being planned. The staff and managers within the initial eight services to introduce ISFs were brought together in a series of workshops in which they were informed about the plans and encouraged to share their opinions as to the overall vision and how to achieve it in practice. These events were also seen as an opportunity to encourage networking between service areas and localities within Choice Support. Participants were therefore put into groups with representatives from other services. This enabled them to learn more about each other's roles and practice, and thereby challenged potential assumptions and stereotyping about other service areas. In addition to these larger events, senior managers met with the operational teams in small groups to enable more in-depth discussions and to symbolise how committed the organisation was to these changes. Training sessions were held with staff and service managers, as many did not fully understand how and what funding people received, and these sessions were followed by regular 'top ups' to enable staff to steadily and readily 'digest' information.

Forums were held with the individuals who used the services to inform them of what was being planned and to enable them to raise any queries. The involvement managers within Choice Support helped with the arrangements of these sessions. If someone had particular communication needs that meant it would be difficult for them to attend group sessions, they were met with individually. Time was also spent informing family members and responding to their concerns.

DIMENSIONS

Dimensions made personalisation an organisational priority and developed a far-reaching strategy that not only stretched into the day-to-day work of support teams, but also included the systems and processes of the supporting departments and structures (see Figure 7.2). Importantly, this was not just a change of process or structure, but one of culture and behaviour as the organisation realised that its 'personality' or 'character' needed to be consistent throughout to succeed. (More details of Dimensions' approach to developing ISFs 'at scale' are given in Chapter 7.) Dimensions aimed to create a feeling of excitement and anticipation (a 'buzz') across the organisation alongside the important features of any successful project, such as developing success criteria, measures, baseline data, timescales and responsibilities. Dimensions invested heavily in a core project team (including those that could act as sounding boards and critical friends from outside the organisation) and developed a comprehensive guide for those taking on this journey locally.

---

2   See www.prosci.com/adkar-model/overview-3, accessed 1 July 2014.

Workshops, quizzes, posters, films and regular e-briefings all added to some very wide-reaching internal communication. All staff were trained in the person-centred thinking skills and tools, and performance coaches were accredited in training in person-centred thinking skills and able to coach support teams across the organisation.

REAL LIFE OPTIONS

A project manager was appointed to oversee the TORCH programme, and to avoid potential duplication or overlap of responsibilities they also took on the role of service manager. Real Life Options set up a high-level internal steering group which included representatives from the board, senior managers, marketing and communication, finance and human resources. A monthly core group was developed in Birmingham which brought together Tunstall, HSA and the University to share progress and problem solve any issues regarding the partnership. The core group then met with the local services managers to undertake a collective reflection each month on what was working and what was not working.

LOOK AHEAD

Look Ahead worked closely with the commissioners for both services in which they have introduced ISFs. The Coventry Road scheme was already in existence and they agreed with the commissioner that existing staffing vacancies could be frozen in order to free up funding to be used on a more flexible basis. This posed some risks for the organisation and the people accessing the service, as reduced staff may have led to people's core needs not being met and to the remaining staff becoming anxious. This is a particular issue in services that support people with complex needs, as it is vital for staff and the individuals to develop a trusting relationship. Monitoring arrangements were put in place to detect if the well-being of the individuals in the service had declined during the pilot. Changes were also made to organisational processes, such as recruitment of staff and financial management, to ensure that the individuals and the service had the freedom to be more creative in what resources and support were accessed. The rehabilitation service was commissioned with ISFs in place, meaning that such flexibilities were embedded from the outset in the staffing structure and organisational processes.

Conclusion

Each of the organisations took their own approach to managing the organisational changes required to implement ISFs. Whilst each one had its unique features and sequencing, there are a number of common elements – good co-ordination though a project lead and a project board, engagement of key external stakeholders through regular communication and if appropriate their membership on the project board, adaption of relevant organisational processes alongside those directly related to care provision and multiple opportunities for staff to find out and engage with the change. In Chapter 7 we learn in more detail about Dimensions' experience of creating an infrastructure for change at scale.

Chapter 7

Creating an Infrastructure for ISFs at Scale

Introduction

Dimensions has been discovering what personalisation means in practice, not just for managers and staff, but for everyone throughout the organisation. Enabling people to have a greater say over the services they receive and a role in the delivery of those services is a central theme of the organisation's values. Dimensions has made personalisation an organisational priority and has developed a far-reaching strategy that not only stretches into the day-to-day work of support teams, but also includes the systems and processes of the organisation's supporting departments and structures. Importantly, Dimensions recognised that this was not just a change of process or structure, but one of culture and behaviour, as the organisation realised that its 'personality' or 'character' needed to be consistent throughout to succeed. This chapter examines how Dimensions is making these changes to the DNA of its organisation.

Building on earlier work

Dimensions has been working steadily to explore the impact of the personalisation agenda in their organisation. In Dimensions' first phase of work, they discovered how the organisation would need to respond to individuals and families having personal budgets, and what it would mean to be able to offer bespoke services to them.[1] This led Dimensions to look at what this same approach could look like if it was used with people that they currently supported, and they learned with Anne-Marie and the people with whom she lived, how the service needed to change for Anne-Marie to have greater choice and control over her service.[2] Dimensions knew that the next stage of the journey would be to apply this learning and principles across the organisation so that each person they support benefits from tailored and personalised services with an Individual Service Fund (ISF).

Dimensions had learned significant lessons from the first two phases of the organisation's work – these highlighted the requirement of a significantly different approach to traditional daily practice and the associated implications for staff deployment and workforce development. In summer 2011 Dimensions started on the third phase of their journey: to implement ISFs at scale, and to make these changes they decided to take a depth-and-breadth approach to change.

A depth-and-breadth approach to change

Dimensions recognised that, at the time (and as continues to be the case), the internal and external environment within which the organisation operates is unpredictable and the sands shift. With that in mind they agreed to take a breadth-and-depth approach to the organisation-wide implementation of personalised services:

---

1   Scown, S. and Sanderson, H. (2010) *Making it Personal: A Provider's Journey from Tradition to Transformation.* Theale: Dimensions.
2   Scown and Sanderson (2010).

- Breadth

  Breadth meant that everyone within the organisation would be supported to use person-centred practices within their roles. Managers would use 'Progress for Providers' to self-assess how they are using the person-centred thinking tools both with themselves and their team. Everyone would consistently use Positive and Productive Meetings[3] (a practical meeting process that ensures that people can listen carefully, think clearly and make effective decisions together) and there would be person-centered supervision for staff and an annual appraisal. They were also working towards everyone they support having an annual person-centred review.

- Depth

  Depth referred to working more closely with three of Dimensions' regions at that time (Tyneside, South – Hampshire and Southampton, West Yorkshire – Wakefield) to implement ISFs.

Dimensions decided to take a whole-organisation, multi-layered approach, supporting their operations directors to set their own targets and pace of change within the context of the agreed critical success factors. Dimensions acknowledged that this would be a five-year plan.

Establishing an implementation team

An implementation team for this stage of the personalisation journey was established in late 2011 with a remit to:

- prepare staff teams for the forthcoming changes

- ensure that person-centred thinking tools and person-centred reviews are routinely used

- use the person-centred thinking tools and practices during the 'personalisation journey'

- have special regard to the learning and development needs of the workforce

- prepare people they support and families for the changes in Dimensions' approach and securing their consent where appropriate

- establish a working partnership with relevant local authorities where there is a recognised interest.

The team met regularly to ensure ongoing review of the implementation (and any associated risks) to account for changing circumstances, dealing with problems and exploiting opportunities. It considered the implications for Dimensions' central support services and made recommendations for any necessary changes. It also ensured that the agreed communication strategy would be implemented and rigorously followed.

Core membership of the implementation team at this stage reflected its responsibilities (Figure 7.1). They knew, however, that other people from across the organisation would be critical, including better practice coaches and performance coaches. The core tasks in their initial plan are given in Table 7.1.

---

3   For descriptions of Positive and Productive Meetings, see: Sanderson, H. and Lepkowsky, M.B. (2014) *Person-Centred Teams.* London: Jessica Kingsley Publishers, p.94.

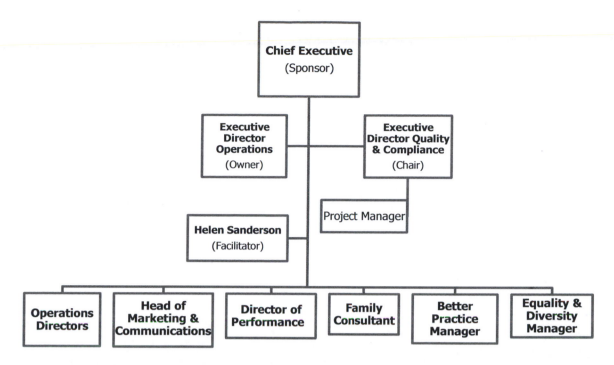

Figure 7.1 Core membership of the Dimensions implementation team

Table 7.1 *Core tasks in the initial plan of the Dimensions implementation team*

Task	Outcome
Identification of internal resource requirements	Establishment of implementation group members and roles
	Agreement on terms of reference for the group
Ensuring that the aims and expectations of the next phase are clearly communicated and available to all involved	A clear communication strategy with graphics that explain how everything fits together
Communication of programme requirements and expectations to all key stakeholders (i.e. people they support, managers and staff, commissioners, families/carers)	Letters to stakeholders involved in programme

cont.

Task	Outcome
Undertaking of sample engagement observations, person-centred thinking assessments and compliance audits	Team support requirements established (including training needs, supervision and appraisal requirements) Detailed programme plan for each location available
Development and implementation of training programme	All staff and key players familiar with person-centred thinking tools and practices
Allocation (i.e. determination of each person's available financial resources, identification of core and individual costs)	Each person will have an agreed allocation of money All core costs will be agreed
Support planning (i.e. each person's support requirements established based on 'perfect weeks' and how best to support them)	Dimensions will know what good support looks like for each person by each having an agreed support plan inclusive of matching people, perfect week, individualised support (rota) arrangements and natural supports
Introduction of individual contracts, support agreements and commitments to all relevant parties	Each person will have an agreed individual contract and support agreement
Implementation (i.e. agreed plans carried out by the person and their support team)	Support delivered as specified by the person. Dimensions' time management system fully utilised (rota planning)
Introduction of person-centred performance management to each person supported, their families/carers and support staff	Each person supported will be fully involved in the ongoing appraisal of support staff (utilising the one-page profile) Each member of staff will have a personal development plan that reflects personal requirements and feedback from people supported

Task	Outcome
Review (i.e. undertaking of engagement observations and person-centred thinking assessments)	Evidence of success and learning
Person-centred review (i.e. undertaking of a person-centred review for each person supported)	Each person will be receiving support as agreed. Dimensions will know what is working and what is not working, and any actions required will be identified
Working Together for Change (i.e. individual reviews inform strategic change)	Will identify barriers and areas not working and inform strategic plans
	Areas of good practice and success stories shared internally and externally

At the early meetings of the implementation team in late 2011 and early 2012, there were some key decisions made as a result of discussions about the practicalities of delivering everything they had set out in the initial plan. This included a recognition that, at the same time as trying to implement this plan, the organisation was undergoing other significant changes, such as a wholesale review of terms and conditions and a challenging operating climate.

Developing a detailed roadmap

The implementation team, in conjunction with their stakeholders, developed a *vision statement* for their personalisation journey. In essence, this is an 'elevator pitch' that they hoped everyone could use when asked the question, 'What is your personalisation journey about?':

> The personalisation journey will enable people they support to have choice and control over what they do, how they spend their time, who supports them and how they are supported. Dimensions' culture and practices are changing, but they will support their staff in using the person-centred thinking tools and techniques to make this happen. Being a person-centred organisation is Dimensions' priority.

The vision statement then became the basis of Dimensions' one-page strategy (Figure 7.2), which also incorporates the organisation's critical success factors. This outlines what success means, how the organisation works to achieve it and how the organisation measures it for people the organisation supports, families, employees and the organisation itself. This has been produced as a laminated poster and appears in Dimensions' offices and workspaces within services.

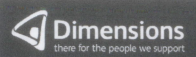 **Dimensions**
there for the people we support

Personalisation: our one page strategy

The Personalisation Journey will enable people we support to have choice and control over what they do, how they spend their time, who supports them and how they are supported. Our culture and practices are changing, but we will support our staff in using the person-centred thinking tools and techniques to make this happen. Being a person-centred organisation is our priority.

Success means...

For the people we support and their families...

They have...
- choice and control in their own lives
- person-centred & flexible schedules
- reduced support hours
- input into the business planning process

They are...
- achieving what they want
- informed in what we do
- connected to strong circles of support
- in paid employment & volunteer posts
- represented at all levels
- involved in staff straining, recruitment and performance management

Families and friends are engaged and involved and along with communities, have a big part to play.

For employees...

All employees ...
- understand and use person-centred thinking tools and techniques
- are trained in person-centred thinking tools
- use person-centred supervision and Dimensions' performance management system
- can articulate and describe what personalised services are
- are motivated by the outcomes for the people we support

Positive and productive meetings are used well and consistently through the organisation.

For the organisation...

Dimensions...
- leads the way
- is seen as radical
- has a person-centred culture
- has a good partnership with local authorities
- has good IT that supports delivery of services

Each person and home has a plan for development of personalised services.

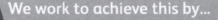
We work to achieve this by...

(For the people we support)
- My support plan
- Decision making agreements
- Person-centred reviews
- Individual Service Fund agreement
- Working together for change
- Relationship map
- Community connections
- Roles & responsibilities
- Important to/for
- Person-centred performance management
- Matching support
- Good day/bad day
- One page profile
- What's working/what's not working.

(For employees)
- Introduction to using person-centred thinking tools training
- Positive & productive meetings
- Person-centred performance management
- Matching support
- Learning logs
- One page profiles
- Roles & responsibilities
- What's working/what's not working
- Working together for change.

(For the organisation)
- Working together for change
- Positive & productive meetings
- One page profile
- What's working/what's not working
- Learning logs
- Roles and responsibilities
- Person-centred performance management
- 4+1 questions.

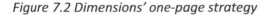
We measure this by...

(For the people we support)
- 100 % people with My support plan that includes:
  - Decision making agreements & actions and Person-centred reviews
  - Person-centred reviews with actions resulting from 'What's working/what's not working'
- 100 % people with signed Individual Service Fund agreements
- [x] people have external circles of support
- [x] people in paid employment
- [x] people volunteering
- [x] attending Everybody Counts meetings
- 100 % induction sessions to involve people we support or families
- 100 % performance management appraisals to involve people we support and families all relevant staff (e.g. Support Workers, Service Managers)
- 100 % recruitment processes to involve people we support.

(For employees)
- 75 % employees who can describe, and share their experience of using 5 x person-centred thinking tools
- 100 % staff training reflects training received on the person-centred thinking tools
- 100 % staff supervised and appraised using the Dimensions performance management system is recorded
- 75 % are able to articulate and describe what personalised services are
- 100 % of staff with one page profiles.

(For the organisation)
- We receive 6 invitations to speak at external events in a year
- 100 % employees engaged in new person-centred performance management system
- 100 % staff completed breadth training person-centred thinking tools
- 100 % services with a Service Improvement Plan
- 100 % people with person-centred reviews
- [X] % of local authorities would recommend us or write a positive reference for us.

Figure 7.2 Dimensions' one-page strategy

Developing further the graphics that had made the first two phases of Dimensions' journey successful, the organisation refined a *personalisation journey map* (Figure 7.3), which helps explain the different stages of the journey. Dimensions has found that these visual interpretations help make the connections for the organisation's employees.

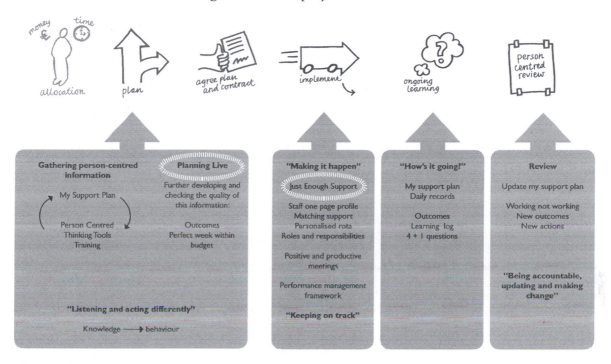

Figure 7.3 Dimensions' personalisation journey map

The map brings all of Dimensions' related planning, practice and review processes together, starting by illustrating how they gather information about a person using person-centred thinking tools and My Support Plan, with both of these processes reinforcing and helping the other. Employees may have come across My Support Plan before receiving training on the person-centred thinking tools; in each case, when they did, the support planning process was greatly enhanced.

The Planning Live process focused teams even further; this is an event where they further develop information from people's support plans, resulting in setting real direction and a timely quality check. All of these processes are designed not only to help increase knowledge, but to change behaviour and culture. The remaining activities on the map illustrate how Dimensions plans to implement what is discovered during Planning Live, using all the tools at hand to embed a positive and productive culture and keep the person at the centre of all the organisation does. Their ongoing learning is facilitated by the use of learning logs and 4+1 reviews that help keep the support plan alive and relevant, culminating in an annual person-centred review process that creates new outcomes and actions which are, in turn, implemented and monitored – holding the support team to account.

Guide and toolkit

Dimensions also developed a guide and toolkit for their personalisation journey for the organisation's regions which was launched on 15 August and 24 September 2012 to members of their leadership group (senior managers) and other service managers and coaches. The guide was very much based around the learning Dimensions had captured during its journey with Anne-Marie, particularly the top tips they had identified. Dimensions set out the approach the organisation felt managers should take when trying to roll this out locally. A toolkit of accompanying templates and documents was made available as an online resource. The steps Dimensions outlined included:

- *Developing a project plan* for delivering personalisation within the organisation's region or service. This needed to address the 'breadth' issues, that is, training and support for staff in embedding the person-centred thinking tools and techniques; and then the 'depth' issues, that is, introducing ISFs for the people Dimensions supports.

- *Establishing a project team* that included representation from operational and resource ring functions (e.g. finance, human resources and performance coach), whose functions, support and input will be critical, as well as considering the involvement of other people (e.g. family members, advocates, the people Dimensions supports) to help the organisation achieve the outcomes required.

- *Communication with stakeholders* to foster the spirit of partnership and co-production. This includes people Dimensions supports and families.

- *Equality impact assessment* to enable the assessment of the implications of decisions and actions.

- *Engagement observations, Progress for Providers assessments and compliance audits* to measure the engagement of meaningful activity of people Dimensions supports and identify team support requirements.

- *Risk assessment and impact assessment* to ensure that any associated risks were considered and that adequate control measures are in place, and to address issues around the impact on people or services of any actions that may be taken.

- *Training programme* so that all staff are familiar with the person-centred thinking tools and practices.

- *Allocation* to determine each person's available resource, what money is in their control to spend and how they can spend it.

- *Planning Live and Just Enough Support* to show how Dimensions planned with the person to identify and implement the outcomes.

- *Introducing ISFs* to reflect the work done and decisions made during support planning.

- *Review* to check progress six months later and evidence success and learning.

Dimensions also produced a glossary for its personalisation journey that is available internally and externally, and identified organisational champions for each aspect of the journey, accessible by anyone across the organisation.

Understanding the baseline

Dimensions wanted all managers to understand their own baseline, and that of their teams, in terms of how well person-centred practices are used, but the organisation also needed to capture its position at a higher level. Dimensions used the Survey Monkey tool to convert the Progress for Providers template into an online survey. Each manager – including not just those within their operations directorate, but also their business support functions – completed this self-assessment with each member of their team in late 2012, and action plans were developed. The managers had the results fed back to them, took ownership of the action plans and have since reviewed it.

Embedding the foundations across the organisation

To fully realise personalisation, Dimensions knew that the process had to be approached and used in a person-centred way. Dimensions had learned in the past that you need to develop and invest in your staff in order for real change to happen. With the range of person-centred thinking tools defining the organisation's personalisation journey, Dimensions invested in nine of its performance coaches to become accredited trainers in person-centred thinking (with the Learning Community for Person-Centred Practices).

The coaches' role was to train, support and coach support teams as they embarked on the journey. Depending on the Progress for Providers assessment, coaches would design a bespoke programme for each service manager and team. To make sure Dimensions was both ambitious and realistic about what the coaches could achieve, the organisation developed their offer and shared it with service managers (one condition was that you had to fill the room during workshops) and teams to:

- weave personalisation into their everyday work

- challenge behaviours and culture

- run a two-day workshop in each region each year (operations directors choose who attends)

- facilitate oneday workshops in the region and follow up with coaching or mentoring (beneficial and more effective if teams go through workshops together)

- use themes in Action Learning Sets

- ensure that staff are trained in facilitating Planning Live.

The coaches have become a vital link for the ongoing need for cultural change in services, a useful and supportive reference point for support teams that provides the guidance needed to continue with the journey.

CHANGING SUPPORT PAPERWORK

By the time the implementation team began to meet, they had seen the start of the roll-out of 'My Support Plan', a new support planning process for use with everyone Dimensions supports. My Support Plan took the place of many different styles and formats of support planning that were being used across the organisation and replaced them with a process that used person-centred thinking (and the related tools) as its heartbeat. My Support Plan is outcome focused and is designed to help people develop a cohesive description of a person, drawing on what is important to someone throughout the process. The language and ethos of Dimensions' personalisation journey fitted neatly together with the new support planning paperwork, and importantly the discoveries for and by a person during the journey adds to and updates the plan.

ASSISTIVE TECHNOLOGY

Dimensions' learning so far told the organisation that assistive technology will play a big part in the personalisation journey, and in particular within the discussions taking place during the 'Just Enough Support' stage. This had been very important when taking the journey with Anne-Marie and her staff team; for example, it raised the question of what technology could increase choice and control for people around the house, such as switches for kitchen equipment and easy-handles for bath taps. It also led to conversations about whether a person requires a waking-night staff or if it is a better option to spend their money on telecare technology that monitors and alerts when necessary.

Of course, all of these decisions must be made with a particular person and set of circumstances in mind, and they are vital to Dimensions achieving the right support for a person based on what is most important to them. Dimensions is very clear that assistive technology must be part of the creative conversation that occurs when figuring out the best way for a person's desired outcomes to be realised according to value for money, what is important to someone, and increasing choice and control.

PERSON-CENTRED THINKING SKILLS

Based on Dimensions' learning from the second phase of the journey with Anne-Marie and her staff team, the organisation knew that having its staff understanding and using person-centred thinking skills would be critical to the success of the rest of the journey. Following some initial planning, however, Dimensions quickly realised that although the organisation would want all of its staff to attend a two-day training course, this would not be affordable or practical. Dimensions considered alternatives to this and made the decision to develop an e-learning course for person-centred thinking, working closely with Helen Sanderson Associates and an e-learning developer. Dimensions knew it was going to take some time to develop such a course; however, in the meantime the organisation did the following:

- Trained the organisation's performance and better practice coaches in person-centred thinking. Through this process, Dimensions was able to train up to 300 of their employees in the initial three regions, and ten coaches gained accreditation with the international learning community.

- Arranged *Positive and Productive Meetings* training for all of the organisation's leadership team and other managers (more than 75 people) for them to cascade to all of their team and other local meetings. This training was also extended to Dimensions' board and committee members.

The person-centred thinking e-learning course was developed through late 2012 and 2013 and went live to Dimensions' employees in August 2013. It covers 12 of the most frequently used person-centred thinking tools within the organisation's approach to support planning and the personalisation journey. The feedback has been very positive. Staff were expected to complete the course within their first 12 weeks of being at Dimensions.

Those staff who work in Dimensions' business support functions are also expected to complete the course. Dimensions provides opportunities and encouragement for every member of its workforce to feel included in the organisation's primary aim of supporting people. This is true even for staff working in the business support departments, who may not be directly supporting people but are in the background setting up a good foundation and infrastructure so Dimensions can do what it does best.

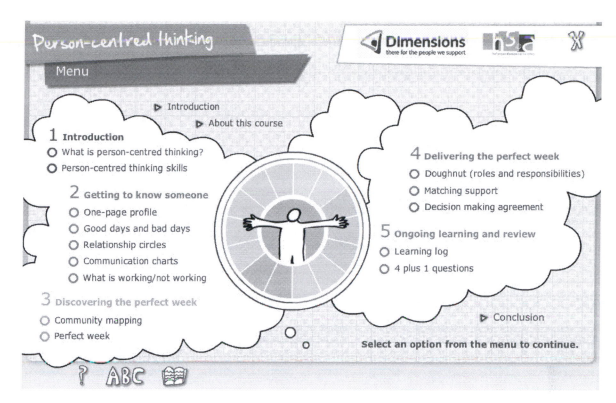

Figure 7.4 Dimensions e-learning course contents

One-page profiles

It was already part of Dimensions' organisational standards that, as well as everyone supported by Dimensions, everyone who works for Dimensions should have a one-page profile. Over these past few years this has been strengthened in their way of working.

All executive team members and board members have their one-page profiles on their website. The majority of staff have their one-page profile on their e-mail signature. One-page profiles are used when meetings with external bodies are being held (e.g. when a group of people supported by Dimensions went to meet MPs, they asked the MPs for their one-page profiles and shared theirs in return). Teams have created one-page profiles for their whole department. One of Dimensions' executive directors wrote a blog about the '101 ways to use a One Page Profile'.[4] Dimensions has produced guidance and tips for staff when developing their own one-page profile.

Monitoring progress

After the guide and toolkit were introduced in autumn 2012, Dimensions asked each regional operations director to work with their managers and teams to develop project plans for rolling out the personalisation journey in their regions. Throughout 2013, Dimensions held 6-weekly conference calls with the operations directors to review progress, discussing things that were working and going well, and things that were not working and whether support or clarification was required. Dimensions also reviewed the measures that are set out in the organisation's one-page strategy. Where a common theme emerged, Dimensions produced guidance notes or newsletters that could be shared across the organisation (Figure 7.5).

---

4   See www.dimensions-uk.org/news-and-events/101-ways-to-use-a-one-page-profile, accessed 1 July 2014.

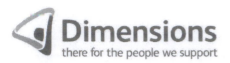
there for the people we support

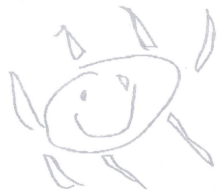

Our Personalisation Journey
Personalisation & Recruitment

Acknowledging and respecting diversity is an integral part of the personalisation journey, and a key point in the recruitment processes.

We use all kinds of person centred thinking tools, such as **one page profile, my history, important to and for, my perfect week, good day/bad day** to collect really useful information that describes who someone is and what is important to them.

The more detailed information we have, the better chance we have of recruiting the right person.

The **matching tool** then helps map the priorities, what's essential, and what's desirable.

Use this information to help inform the job description (for support worker and Lead Support Worker roles only) and person specification for the person we support.

See overleaf for tips on how & when to recruit and shortlisting & selection

Things we can't do

Equality legislation means we cannot say we want to recruit someone from a particular country but we can say we need them to be able to speak a particular language, or share the same cultural values or beliefs.

Equally, we can't say that we want to recruit someone of a particular age but we can ask for people who share a particular interest or hobby.

We do from time to time use GOR (genuine occupational requirement) when it is necessary to recruit only male or female employees.

If you are not sure, then please contact a member of the recruitment team who will be happy to advise

Figure 7.5 Dimensions' guidance notes and newsletter

Embedding quality systems and approaches

The most dramatic change to Dimensions quality systems has been informed by the organisation's personalisation journey one-page strategy. Dimensions wanted to make sure that what the organisation 'sees as good' has its derivative in personalising services and support, and helping to increase choice and control. Each regional managing director has a regional plan to ensure that the personalisation journey is being pursued in line with organisational expectations and time frame. It is the responsibility of each locality manager to drive these plans forward and ensure that each person they support will have an ISF by 2016.

Dimensions' quality-of-life statements come from what people the organisation supports have been telling them is important through Working Together For Change, a process that gathers together all the information that people Dimensions supports have been reporting through their person-centred reviews. Dimensions measures its performance against these statements, which in turn may well change in time depending on what people say is most important to them.

Dimensions' challenge is to measure the success of the organisation's processes in providing the opportunity for great outcomes, and Dimensions' own outcomes against what people have told them they want in life. That is why Dimensions is making new changes to further focus the organisation's auditing procedures on outcomes related to quality of life and increasing choice and control.

Changing systems and process

How Dimensions approaches allocation is described in Chapter 2. The other significant system changes were in relation to Dimensions' time management system (DTMS) to help managers plan rotas as well as how they manage performance and recruitment.

THE DIMENSIONS TIME MANAGEMENT SYSTEM

The DTMS provides the facility to schedule the support requirements of the people that Dimensions supports, and to assign the most appropriate available staff to satisfy those requirements. The application is accessible to all managers and provides them with relevant person-specific information. The DTMS provides a facility to show a planned schedule, and the actual support delivered, and electronically passes authorised information into the payroll system, eliminating the need for central timesheet processing and reducing invoice-process complexity. The DTMS provides managers with tools to manage their staff teams, including setting and monitoring training requirements, against staff skills. It is, essentially, a very efficient way of building Dimensions' support around people it supports and according to the organisation's chosen activities and best-matched support.

At the heart of great support is a focus on meaningful involvement in valued activities and relationships. For this to happen, a person usually requires the best support possible, tailored to a particular situation and set of circumstances. For example, if someone requires the upmost focus and concentration whilst shopping in a busy supermarket, it may be best that they be supported by someone who is calm, organised, resists the urge to speak too frequently and is available to support the person at times when the shop is less busy. The kind of information that is best gathered through using one-page profiles and the matching tool can be turned into schedules and diaries by using the DTMS: just enter an activity, a time and a person that is a good match.

PERFORMANCE MANAGEMENT

With increasing demand on Dimensions internally and externally, to get things right it is important that the organisation be able to demonstrate the standard of work and the achievement of its employees. Dimensions needed a performance management system that gets to the heart of how well the organisation's employees are performing in their role and the contribution they make.

At the end of 2012, Dimensions introduced a revised system in preparation for the organisation's 2013 appraisal season. The revised system uses the person-centred thinking tools, as they are at the centre of everything Dimensions does, from planning with people the organisation supports through to supporting its employees in their employment.

At one-to-one supervision, core tasks are discussed based on what is working and what is not working in order to explore work, contribution and consider areas to celebrate. Annual appraisals use the 4+1 person-centred thinking tool to capture involvement and contribution throughout the year. Prior to the meetings, managers also capture feedback from a sample of people who work closely with the employee; that may include family members, people the organisation supports and other professionals.

RECRUITMENT AND SELECTION

Dimensions has produced a guide related to the personalisation journey in the context of recruitment and selection. This outlines the useful approaches and tools that are necessary when recruiting the best-matched staff to people Dimensions supports. During support planning each person asks questions about two main areas: 'How do I want to live my life?' and 'How do I want to be supported (and who supports me)?' Dimensions needs the answers to both of these questions in order to be confident of recruiting the right person. Only by getting a true description of what is important to people about how they want to live will Dimensions get a good picture of what support they need and who is best to carry it out. The aim is to build on the important (yet limiting for most people) first steps of including people on interview panels by integrating a person-centred approach at every stage of the recruitment process. The guide explains how this is done, including: developing a person-centred job description; a description of what the best-matched staff must be (person specification); personalising the advert and thinking of the best place to advertise by looking at the 'Community Connections' section of the person's support plan; including the person and/or family in the interview; and asking candidates to complete their own one-page profile.

COMMUNICATING DIMENSIONS' PERSONALISATION JOURNEY

As Dimensions' implementation phase was underway, it tried to create a feeling of excitement and anticipation (a 'buzz') across the organisation. Dimensions used some of the documents referred to above – the one-page strategy, briefing notes and so forth – but the organisation supplemented this by providing quizzes for managers to use with their teams, short films about the journey and articles in the organisation's staff newsletters to be as wide-reaching as possible.

Dimensions has also produced an 'easy read' guide for people the organisation supports and documentation specifically for families. Dimensions uses social media: the organisation set up a blog to chart the personalisation journey, which incorporates the experience of family members, and it uses Twitter to talk about the personalisation journey. Each member of the leadership group made three pledges related to Dimensions' personalisation journey and what they would do to contribute. Managers within the regions engaged their staff teams in different ways. Their top tips to create a buzz about the personalisation journey are as follows:

- Put up posters and pictures of the person-centred thinking tools in the office to keep reminding people about them.

- Invite the family consultants to your regional meetings to bring the experience to life from a family perspective.

- Ask each member of staff to make a pledge about the personalisation journey, and share this with colleagues; incorporate these into performance management and the regional strategy, and review progress.

- Ask staff teams to give presentations to their managers and the regional project team about personalisation and their understanding of it. (People have done this using different formats, such as video, PowerPoint, role play and so forth.)

- Bring staff from different teams together for discussions and workshops to share experiences and different perspectives.

- Include family members, local commissioners and other external people as members on regional personalisation project teams.

- Use the 'Family Charter' as a catalyst for involvement and to help develop circles of support.

- Use the 'Personalisation Guide' as the agenda for the meetings, separating out the sections as key topics for discussion.

- Split the book *Making it Personal for Everyone* (by Steve Scown and Helen Sanderson) into chapters, and read and discuss them at team meetings, like in a book group.

- Hold 'team days' as an introduction or refresher to the tools before the personalisation journey begins.

- Give every member of staff a printout of the one-page strategy.

- Build into the process a point at which the team can hear a few months post-implementation how things have changed for people the organisation supports.

- Talk about personalisation to remind staff for what they are there: they can make a difference to people by delivering personalised support that improves people's quality of life.

Dimensions' learning

Dimensions' staff all needed to change together. There have been many reports of staff 'getting it' and embracing the change towards personalised services. Certainly, the person-centred thinking tools are now widespread in their use, with support plans exploring not what they should do for someone, but who they are, what they find precious in life and how they want to live. Staff are learning that what they do has to take the lead from such questions and that standing still is not an option. Late in 2013, Dimensions carried out a 'lessons learned' review of the organisation's personalisation journey to date. These are some of the early lessons about what is working and what is not working:

- Changes in relation to people Dimensions supports:

  ○ services designed specifically for the people Dimensions supports

  ○ greater accessibility to activities and community opportunities

- more choice and control in their lives
- confidence to voice their opinions
- Dimensions' personalisation journey is 'bringing their dreams to life'.

- Changes in relation to staff:
  - confidence and enthusiasm to be creative
  - more reflective about how their support influences the lives of the people Dimensions supports
  - a deeper understanding of what personalisation really is
  - embedded in what staff are doing day-to-day
  - empowered to check up on each other and point out what could be improved upon.

- Changes in relation to Dimensions as an organisation:
  - promotion of positive working partnerships with local authorities and commissioners
  - enhanced views of Dimensions on the part of external partners
  - challenging traditional-based services with a real tangible solution – the personalisation journey
  - live and current personalisation about which everybody knows
  - commissioners: Dimensions 'gets it' and is 'forward thinking'.

- What is driving creativity:
  - outstanding and inspiring individuals at every level
  - staff buying into the principles of personalisation
  - having the personalisation tools and guidance available
  - understanding local resources (no one size fits all)
  - celebrating creativity motivates others
  - making personalisation high on the agenda.

- How Dimensions could learn better from each other's innovative practices:
  - asking 'how did you do that?' so it can be replicated
  - capturing and sharing success stories and good-practice ideas
  - personalisation newsletter
  - road shows
  - get people together and conversation flowing
  - at regional and national levels
  - a more rapid sharing process
  - giving all staff a chance to voice their creative practice.

- Key factors in success so far:
  - getting key players on board and selling the personalisation journey
  - flexible and available staff
  - the quality of the toolkit and training
  - having local authorities on board
  - engaging with the people Dimensions supports from the very first conversation
  - momentum
  - a regional plan with actions and timescales
  - insisting all staff read the book and evidence their understanding
  - regularly assessing motivation
  - quarterly workshops
  - teams receiving feedback
  - the phased approach
  - keeping it fun and engaging.
- Challenges and difficulties:
  - not having enough time to devote to the journey
  - how to be creative when there is no money
  - keeping up motivation during challenging circumstances
  - lack of understanding
  - families
  - support workers
  - councils
  - external funders
  - e-learning and 'easy read' materials not being available at the start of the personalisation journey
  - finding alternative housing solutions
  - services starting the personalisation journey from very different places
  - change to regional boundaries.

Conclusion

Dimensions believes that it will be a five-year journey to introduce ISFs to everyone, and the organisation is part of the way there. Taking a depth-and-breadth approach means that the impact of change will be felt by everyone (the breadth) whilst learning continues about what it takes to ensure that ISFs are able to profoundly change the opportunities and experiences of each person who holds an ISF (the depth). In Chapter 8 we learn from another organisation, Real Life Options, about how they approached supporting their managers.

Chapter 8

Supporting Managers

Introduction

The support that managers receive to implement Individual Service Funds (ISFs) is crucial to ensure that ISFs result in people having greater choice and control in their lives. Each of the organisations provided managers with training and support in a variety of ways, including training in person-centred approaches and practices, direct 'on the job' coaching, mentoring and support through Action Learning Sets. In this chapter we focus on the process used by Real Life Options (RLO) to support managers in the first year of their ISF implementation.

Going beyond training

All of the organisations provided training for their managers, and most of them provided additional support to ensure that managers were able to implement the practical and cultural changes the ISFs require. Dimensions supported managers through externally facilitated Action Learning Sets and providing individual mentoring and support to regional managers given by the ex-CEO of another provider organisation who had direct experience of developing ISFs himself. Other organisations, for example, Certitude, also provided their managers with support from a consultant with expertise in ISFs. He provided problem-solving support as well as support for the direction and pace of the project. Lisa, the manager at Bruce Lodge, received on-site support and coaching to facilitate the one-page profile meetings, and to support the practical implementation and cultural changes within the home.

At RLO, in the first year of implementation, the manager's team had a combination of training, problem-solving workshops and direct coaching to use Planning Live as well as Just Enough Support. The staff and managers had come to work for RLO as part of a TUPE[1] transfer. A senior manager from RLO supported them, and staff undertook some training in person-centred approaches as part of supporting them to work with RLO and their commitment to person-centred practices. The senior manager left and a new project manager replaced her to manage the project of delivering ISFs overall and to act as the local service manager.

Preparation

The process of supporting the managers began with preparation, updating and improving their one-page profiles, taking stock of their existing knowledge and skills in person-centred practices and understanding the 'road map' of the journey they were going to take. From this understanding of where they were, and what they needed to do, they co-designed their training and support programme with the consultant.

---

1   TUPE refers to the Transfer of Undertakings (Protection of Employment) Regulations 2006 as amended by the Collective Redundancies and Transfer of Undertakings (Protection of Employment) (Amendment) Regulations 2014. The TUPE rules apply to organisations of all sizes and protect employees' rights when the organisation or service they work for transfers to a new employer.

DEVELOPING ONE-PAGE PROFILES

We all know that attending training is not the same as being able to competently use a new skill in practice. Implementing ISFs requires managers to be confident and competent in using person-centred practices as a habit, in their day-to-day role as managers, and supporting and coaching their team.

The previous year, leaders in RLO had worked on creating internal best practice standards for one-page profiles (Figure 8.1). These standards had not been used in the training that managers had received, and the managers were unfamiliar with them. Although managers already had one-page profiles, not surprisingly, they did not reflect RLO's standards. As it was important that all staff had one-page profiles that reflected RLO's standards, it was crucial to start with managers and making sure that their one-page profiles reflected best practice.

The initial work with managers was to support them to review and improve their one-page profiles, and to use Progress for Providers to establish their existing knowledge, skills and ability to apply person-centred practices to their role.

USING PROGRESS FOR PROVIDERS: ESTABLISHING WHERE THE MANAGERS ARE STARTING FROM

Progress for Providers is an established self-assessment tool with which managers rate themselves against a range of statements, where five represents best practice. The managers spent half a day with a consultant to explore examples of what best practice is (i.e. what a score of four or five would look like) and to support them to accurately rate themselves. The overall scores were mainly two and three.

HAVING A ROAD MAP

In order to support the managers to prepare for their journey, they were given a comprehensive document that effectively was the road map to implementing ISFs based on the model developed with Dimensions. Each of the managers was also given a copy of *Making it Personal* by Steve Scown and Helen Sanderson which describes their experience of trying to implement ISFs with six individuals. Although RLO was planning to use ISFs with over 90 people, the principles and the process was the same.

CO-DESIGNING A PROGRAMME OF TRAINING AND SUPPORT FOR MANAGERS

The managers met with a consultant to co-design a training and support programme that reflected where they were and the road map of the journey. Alongside this there was a day each month for the managers to come together with the project team to review progress and problem-solve together. The support programme for managers included some very specific training on Just Enough Support and Planning Live, and how to make changes to meetings and rotas; however, the programme focused primarily on coaching and supporting managers directly.

One Page Profiles

What is a one page profile?
Quite simply a one page profile tells us about you as a person. It tells people what others like and admire about you; what is important to you and how to support you well.

Why do we have them?
So that we know what is important to each of us and how to support each other.
Each of us have gifts and talents; we all will have things that are very important to us and we will have unique support requirements. One page profiles help us to share this information with others, our families/friends, direct support, managers and colleagues so that we can get to know each other better and support each other well.

One page profile	What this section is	What this section is not
What people like and admire about me..........	What are your gifts and talents? What do others value about you? What are the positive contributions that you make?	A list of accomplishments or awards – instead it is a summary of your positive characteristics.
What is important to me.........	This tells people in your own words what is really important to you, what your hobbies and interests are, who is important to you and what makes a 'good' day for you.	Simply a list of things you like – instead it is a summary of what really matters to you.
How best to support me.............	What do others need to know to make sure you get the best support possible?	A list of very general hints – instead it is the specific information that would be useful for other people to know about to make sure you feel supported.

How are they developed?
Developing a one page profile can be something you do on your own but often it is best to ask others to contribute. It can be developed with family, friends, your manager, with other team members, people you support, people who support you.

Figure 8.1 RLO's standards for one-page profiles

Learning from the managers: What was working and not working for them?

Every month the managers had a 90-minute meeting with the project team and the consultant to look at the previous month together and reflect on what had worked, what had not worked and what was important for the future. 'Important for the future' was taken to mean what needed to happen in the next month for the programme to progress. This 'working and not working' was done from different perspectives. Each manager wrote, from their perspective, what was working and not working, and important for the future, on separate coloured cards. The project team did the same. This information was then clustered, that is, organised to look at all of the 'working' from the managers' perspectives, cluster them together into themes and give them a title. Then the same process was carried out using the project team's perspective (i.e. looking at what was working from their perspectives as well). This process was repeated for what was not working, and what was important for the future, within the next month.

Once information was clustered and named, each person had an opportunity to comment and reflect. This gave an important opportunity to see where there were similarities and differences between the manager's perspective and the project team's perspective. It was a powerful way of acknowledging the progress the managers were making, and for them to have an opportunity to see this collectively.

Naturally, most of the time was spent on looking at what was not working and identifying the root causes of problems, and what was needed to change them. Some problems were relatively simple to figure out. For example, something that was not working was the managers finding time with the staff to type up the staff's one-page profiles. The project manager offered additional administrative support to make that possible.

Other problems were bigger challenges. What follows are two examples of issues that were identified through clustering what was not working, and how the team addressed these issues. The first issue was 'communicating the process to staff'. Managers said that they were finding it hard to help staff understand the process and what this meant to them. The second issue was 'staff doing their own one-page profiles'. The third issue was that some of the staff had some reluctance and negativity around assistive technology and how that was going to work. (We describe that in Chapter 9, 'Assistive Technology'.)

The afternoon following the session was specifically to spend time with the managers and the project team leader to action and address what was not working, and do some detailed work together. Below are descriptions of how this process worked for two of the problems identified above.

COMMUNICATING THE PROCESS TO STAFF

Managers said that they were finding it difficult to explain what was going to happen during the ISF process, and what that meant for staff. The consultant used the following processes with the managers to help address this:

- co-creating a high-level graphic

- using a card-based game to reinforce the sequence of the process

- an exercise to help managers see which person-centred practice would be used where in the process.

To start, the group created a high-level graphic representation of the process to show what that would look like for four individuals who lived together. (Lickey Hills are local to where the managers were working, so they called the house 'Lickey Hills Way'.) Figure 8.2 shows the step-by-step journey for one individual, and this included what staff would be required to do, and what the individuals would experience for each step of the process.

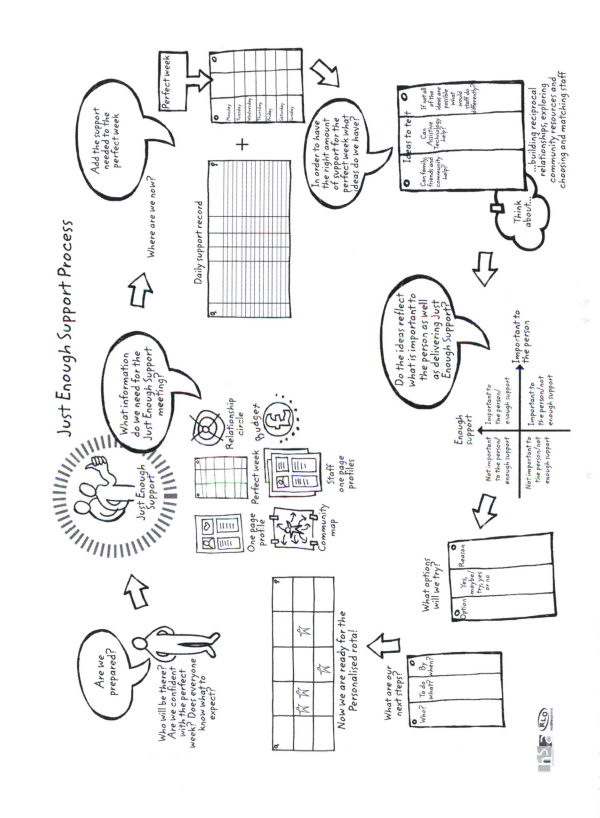

Figure 8.2 High-level graphic shows the ISF process

The first step represented in the graphic is for the individual to know how much money or time they have allocated to them, and to make sure the individual's one-page profile is up to date and accurate. Then the individual is supported to think about who they want to invite to the Planning Live process. Next Planning Live takes place and results in a first-draft description of how the person wants to live – their 'perfect week'. Then the team uses Just Enough Support to understand how to deliver the perfect week within budget and thinks about the role of assistive technology in delivering the perfect week. The process is then to match staff to what the person wants to do during their perfect week. This is why staff one-page profiles are required.

All of this information (how the person wants to live as described in their perfect week and the staff support they need to achieve that) is then put into a personalised rota. After six months, the person reviews how they are living their life, and RLO accounts for how they are spending the person's budget. The person-centred review results in information in the one-page profile being updated, possible changes to who supports the person in their perfect week and what that would mean for the rota.

A poster of the graphic was designed and printed within two weeks, and each manager had a large version of it to put on their office wall. They could then put a 'We Are Here' sticker on it to show where they were with that process for people who lived there.

Card-based game

Key to managers being able to explain the process well to staff was for them to have a deep understanding of the process – the sequence of what happened when, and how person-centred practices would be used. To help the managers consolidate their understanding, the consultant produced a card set where there was a different card for each stage of the process (i.e. Allocation, Plan, Agree, Implement, Ongoing Learning, Review), and on each of those cards was an image that represented that stage. The consultant divided the managers into two groups, shuffled the cards, gave each group of managers a set of the cards and asked them to put them in the order of the process. That was interesting and important to do, as it illustrated that the managers needed further support to be able to do this easily. The most important aspect of this exercise is that it created an opportunity to describe and look at questions around why each of the steps happened in that sequence, and what happened during that process, so we could make sure the managers were really clear about it. Each of the managers had their own set of cards to replicate that process with the staff team to help them understand the process and the sequence. It was a fun activity to do for 30 minutes in a team meeting.

Which person-centred practice is used when?

The third process that the group used was to help the managers understand how the different person-centred thinking tools would be used throughout the whole process of developing ISFs. Again, the consultant used a pack of cards that had each of the person-centred thinking tools on them, and used the big graphic process map the managers working with the consultant had developed together. Each manager was dealt a card (i.e. a person-centred tool) and placed that card somewhere on the process map to indicate that was where they thought that person-centred thinking tool would be used. Then the consultant and the manager had a discussion about which person-centred thinking tool was most appropriate for which part of the process. Naturally, this was drilling down beyond the high-level explanation of the process and the sequence of the cards to how we were going to make that happen and which particular person-centred thinking tools would we find useful at which stage. (Again, these cards were produced for each of the managers to be able to use with their teams to be able to explain where the different person-centred thinking tools fit into the process, and why they were important.)

These three approaches were designed to help managers both, be able to explain well to their staff the process for developing ISFs and to build their own confidence in the sequence and process. By providing the managers with card-based exercises to use with their staff in team meetings, managers had a wider range of ways to help staff understand the process.

MOTIVATING STAFF TO DEVELOP THEIR OWN ONE-PAGE PROFILES

Another example of something that was not working from managers' perspectives over the course of their monthly meetings was to effectively encourage and motivate staff to develop their own one-page profiles. It is very important that staff have detailed one-page profiles that reflect the RLO best practice standards in order for the matching process to be successful. When the individual has developed their perfect week through Planning Live, and the team is looking at how to deliver Just Enough Support, the staff's one-page profiles are required to match staff members, based on their interests and passions, to what the person wants to do (as described in their perfect week). If there is not enough information in the staff one-page profiles that describes what matters to staff members, and what their passions and interests are, it will be impossible to do that part of the process.

Another purpose of having staff create one-page profiles is so that staff are supported well by their managers. If the third section of the one-page profile, which describes 'what good support looks like for me' was done in a very detailed way to give managers enough information about how to support each staff member individually, staff may not always get the personalised support they need so as to be able to deliver ISFs and the cultural change this requires.

To think about how managers can motivate staff to develop their one-page profiles, the group looked at the question, 'If we have to sell one-page profiles to staff, what do we think the potential benefits could be?' What resulted was another graphic (Figure 8.3) with eight benefits of one-page profiles for staff which managers could use to explain to them why they would benefit from doing a one-page profile.

Frequently asked questions with answers

Spending time with the managers in the morning and the afternoon looking at what was working and not working, and important for the future, generated a list of questions managers had about the process – both what was happening now and going forward, to what was coming soon. Each month, the group listed these 'frequently asked questions' (FAQs) and answered them together with the project lead. Immediately after the meeting, these questions were typed and circulated to the managers and updated the following month. This was sent out within a week after every meeting and meant that managers had their difficult questions answered and felt more equipped to communicate this with staff.

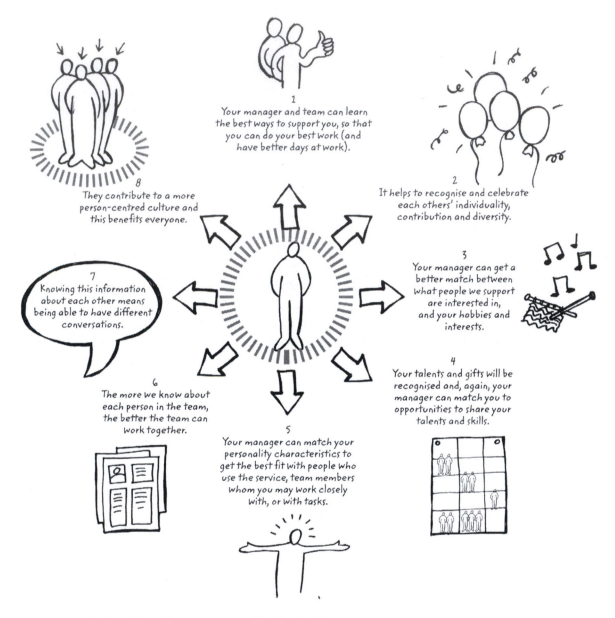

Figure 8.3 The benefits of one-page profiles for staff

Training and coaching managers

Alongside the monthly full-day meeting with managers looking at what was working and not working, and important for the future, and then doing specific work around that in the afternoon, the managers also had a programme of training, coaching and support that was closely connected to this regimen. This was to support the managers to eventually become competent at facilitating Planning Live and Just Enough Support, and to become confident in being able to use person-centred reviews. The whole design of the programme was around skilling up managers and developing their competence and confidence in using these processes to deliver ISFs, and most importantly, to support managers to implement these processes.

PLANNING LIVE

An example of how this worked was Planning Live. The first stage was managers going on a two-day training to understand the Planning Live process: what happened step by step, what was expected from them, the key elements of facilitating this and the resources available. The next step was for each manager to have an opportunity to attend and support a Planning Live session that was being externally facilitated, and then co-facilitate a Planning Live session with a trainer, and then co-facilitate their own Planning Live session. Using this process involved scaffolding the competence and confidence of the managers by first making sure they fully understood the process and then giving them an opportunity to see it happening and to be part of coaching and supported; to co-facilitate it with somebody who had more experience than they did; and to facilitate it with a colleague as well.

Alongside that, each manager had a clear process manual and quality standards they went through with the project manager, who then took responsibility for reviewing progress for Planning Live with the managers in supervision, and making sure the information and the standards met the required expectations.

As well as having specific training, coaching and support, and good materials around key processes such as Planning Live and Just Enough Support, the other opportunity managers had was to think about how to embed these cultural changes within their practice. They were supported to think about what ISFs mean for their role as manager. For example, what does this mean for the way managers run and facilitate meetings with staff? What does this mean for the way the rota gets written, and what are the pros and cons around different ways of doing that? What does it mean for our paperwork and the way we are recording sessions?

Throughout this process managers were supported in different ways and at different levels. They had an opportunity to share what was working and not working, and important for the future; an opportunity to do some problem-solving together on what was not working; an ongoing record of their FAQs and the answers to them; specific training, coaching and support around the processes they needed to learn to put into practice; and support to think about the cultural changes this whole process required.

Personal story: The ISF change process

Bob Timmins, service manager at RLO, describes his experience of the ISF change process:

> As an incredibly busy service manager, the initial thought of managing a large-scale change such as this filled me with dread. Within our sector we are increasingly having budgets squeezed and experiencing larger workloads as a result, and at this point we were an already-depleted management team, and we had also lost our line manager, who was replaced with the project manager, which represented a significant change for the management team.
>
> Having spent time with Sarah (my colleague at RLO), Helen (Helen Sanderson Associates), Robin (Birmingham University) and Kevin (Tunstall), I found that my initial feelings regarding the project had changed: I felt incredibly positive and confident regarding the changes. I believe the main reason for this was seeing how the change to ISFs would not only have financial benefits for the organisation, but more importantly, they would have a direct and positive effect upon the people we support, giving them a choice and control in their lives that I have not experienced previously in my role.

The management team took part in 'working and not working' sessions along with the above core project group and later in sessions with just Helen. These groups were extremely valuable. I found that my colleagues and I had similar concerns and problems to overcome, and whilst we would leave these sessions knowing that we had a lot of work to do, we had a plan and a direction, and we devised graphics, FAQs and revised our plans going forward in relation to Planning Live and involving our teams, people who use our services and family members in the project to help ensure its success.

Here is our main learning on engaging and supporting managers:

- Don't assume that because people have attended training that they are using person-centred practices and are confident and competent. Find out where managers are starting from using Progress for Providers.

- Design supports for managers based on both where they are now (Progress for Providers) and what will be required of them to deliver ISFs.

- Have ways to regularly hear from managers regarding what is working and not working for them, and show that you are acting on this.

- Understand what managers need to be able to implement the next steps in the process (important for the future).

- Act quickly on the issues that managers raise that are getting in the way.

- Keep an ongoing, updated list of FAQs and answers.

- Invest in coaching managers and problem-solving, not just training.

Conclusion

Implementing ISFs requires both investing in, and hearing from, managers. Organisations need to go beyond hearing as well, to being able to quickly act on what managers are telling them is getting in the way as well as celebrating and sharing successes. One of the areas that challenged managers in terms of supporting their staff was assistive technology, and in Chapter 9 we share what Choice Support and RLO tried and learned in implementing assistive technology.

Chapter 9

Assistive Technology

Introduction

Assistive technology has traditionally been used to support older people to live independently; however, there has been increasing interest from care providers in trying to use these technologies within a residential care setting, with a range of people. In this chapter we focus on the experiences of Choice Support and Real Life Options as they sought to deploy the technology at scale alongside the introduction of ISFs. We begin with a short overview of what is meant by 'assistive technology'.

Assistive technology

Assistive technology is any product or service designed to enable independence for disabled and older people. This definition was developed at an assistive technology industry event in 2001 and highlights that the term potentially includes a wide range of different equipment and support. The Foundation of Assistive Technology[1] adds further criteria in its definition – the adoption and use of the technology that is under some measure of control by the end user and there is a level of meaningful interaction by the end user with the product or system. Within health and social care services in the UK, the term is often used in connection with 'telecare' and 'telehealth' in particular. Both of these terms are also broad, with telecare applications ranging from a responsive alarm service, through which a person can summon assistance, to the use of sensors and other detectors to monitor key aspects of a person's situation. This commonly includes detecting if the individual has fallen, opened doors or is at risk from a fire or gas leak. The information gathered is relayed to a support centre which monitors these aspects of the person's well-being and intervenes if they appear to be in danger. Telehealth uses a similar process in relation to people's physical or mental health, through monitoring general vital signs such as blood pressure or those connected with a particular condition such as blood sugar levels in diabetes. The technology can also be used to enable clinicians to undertake virtual consultations rather than rely on a home visit or ask the person to visit their clinic.[2]

ASSISTIVE TECHNOLOGY AND ISFS

The commissioners of the residential care homes provided by the services of Choice Support and Real Life Options required them to find savings from the block contract. One of the major costs within their residential care budgets was employing staff to provide waking-night support. These staff members were undertaking a variety of maintenance and housekeeping tasks during their shifts, but their main purpose was to monitor the well-being of the people living there. Commonly this related to risks connected with epileptic seizures, discomfort due to enuresis or determining that someone was putting themselves or other people in danger through being outside of their bedroom. All of these tasks are essentially connected with monitoring someone's well-being or situation, and rather than staff routinely checking on the individuals, this could be

---

1   See www.fastuk.org.
2   See www.telecare.org.uk for more information regarding telecare and telehealth.

potentially carried out through assistive technology. This would enable the waking-night staff to be replaced with sleep-in staff who could be woken up if someone needed assistance.

Alongside the reduction in staffing costs, both organisations also believed that the introduction of assistive technology could lead to a better quality of life for these individuals. Bedrooms are generally seen as private spaces, and most of us do not appreciate someone coming into this space whilst we are asleep. People in these (and many other) care homes did not have a choice if they wanted someone to come into their bedroom at night, as this was seen as essential to maintaining their health and safety. Having one's bedroom door opened periodically can also lead to a disrupted night's sleep, which can affect mood and overall well-being. This is a particular concern regarding people with behaviours that others find challenging. Assistive technology therefore also provided an opportunity for the organisations to improve quality of life at night and during the day.

What Choice Support tried and learned

Colin, Teresa and Jake's story

Colin, Teresa and Jake live at Blithely House. Their home used to be a registered care home on the former block contract in Southwark. Waking-night provision had been set up in the home for a person who had moved out in 2008. Colin had frequent seizures, but they occurred mainly during the day with 'only' seven at night. All of his seizures were of short duration and he recovered without any need for medication. Apart from his epilepsy, Colin seemed to sleep well and was at very low risk of pressure sores. Teresa slept well through the night and there were no reports of activity or support needs at night. She had incontinence pads in place which were working well. She had been diagnosed with epilepsy but had not had seizures for five years. Jake generally slept well. He was independent and fully mobile. He would occasionally go into the lounge at night, but he could do this without support. Jake could eat raw things from the fridge but this had not happened over the previous 12 months.

The risks were identified as being that Colin could have a seizure at night that would require staff support. Both Colin's and Teresa's skin could become sore due to night-time incontinence. Jake might eat raw food from the fridge or an emergency might occur at night that required staff assistance. The risks were managed by installing an epilepsy alarm for Colin, to alert staff to any seizure, that had a sound monitor fitted which would alert staff if he was vocalising. Colin was also referred for vagus nerve stimulation therapy (VNS), which could reduce or possibly stop his seizures. VNS uses a pulse generator to send mild electrical stimulations to the vagus nerve with the aim of reducing the number, length and severity of seizures. Both Colin and Teresa were referred to a specialist continence advisor to advise if their incontinence pads were the most effective solution. A door sensor was fitted on the kitchen door to alert staff if Jake went into the kitchen at night.

INTRODUCING THE TECHNOLOGY

To identify if technology could potentially have a role in relation to the care of the individuals living in the home, Choice Support needed to assess each individual's requirements during the night-time period. Comprehensive risk assessments were undertaken in which all of the night-time records regarding activities, accidents and incidents over the previous 12 months were closely examined. This enabled the management team to understand the support that each person required at night, the need or type of situation to which this related and the level of risk that this need or situation entailed.[3]

Choice Support decided not to involve a specialised assistive technology company; instead, the service manager and the housing officer researched potential equipment with one of the main criteria being that it would be practical for staff who work in the home to use. Purchasing stand-alone devices also meant there would not be ongoing charges from the supplier. They were bought at relatively low costs of £90 for the sound monitor and £250 for the kitchen door sensor. Spare equipment was also purchased so that they could be replaced in an emergency and spare sets of batteries in case of a power cut.

Assessing for, and purchasing of, the equipment was only the first stage, however, as Choice Support recognised that introducing this equipment and adapting the staffing accordingly would require a significant change process (see Box 9.1). The regional manager proactively engaged with the affected staff members on an individual and group basis to ensure that they were aware of what was being considered and the thinking behind the changes. These discussions also gave the staff members the opportunity to raise their concerns for the individuals living in the service and their own employment. Staff members who were no longer required to work as waking-night staff were either redeployed or offered a generous redundancy package. The regional manager and service managers also discussed the proposals with the individuals within the services and their families.

Box 9.1 Elements of change in introducing assistive technology.

In introducing assistive technology, the elements of change are as follows:

- change in staff numbers and how they are deployed

- change in role of staff and, therefore, potentially skills

- change in support for service users (and potential anxiety of family in connection with this change)

- change process for staff and the potential for resistance to these changes being introduced.

(Adapted from Ellis and Sines)[4]

IMPACT OF ASSISTIVE TECHNOLOGY

The evaluation of the telecare initiative by Choice Support assessed the impact of the changes in relation to its three principle aims: to reduce costs, maintain safety and enhance the quality of the service. (See Chapter 12 for more information regarding the evaluation.)

The following summarises the impacts at Blithely House.

---

3   For further information regarding the deployment of assistive technology by Choice Support, see: Ellis, R. and Sines, D. (2012) *Better Nights: Evaluation of Choice Support in Southwark*. Sheffield: Choice Support.

4   Ellis and Sines (2012) p.20.

> ## Collin, Teresa and Jake's story: Impact of assistive technology
>
> The introduction of the assistive technology meant that the waking-night provision could be replaced with a sleep-in member of staff, as the equipment would alert the person sleeping in on the most pressing issues. There was also an-out-of-hours on-call system for staff to contact a manager in an emergency. Two years on, Blithely House is a much more homely place at night with far less disturbance for Colin, Teresa and Jake. They are all getting a better night's sleep and there have been no serious incidents. There was also an-out-of-hours on-call system for staff to contact a manager in an emergency. Two years on, Blithely House is a much more homely place at night with far less disturbance for Colin, Teresa and Jake. They are all getting a better night's sleep and there have been no serious incidents.

Cost reduction

Throughout 2010–2011 the annual costs of providing support at night for the 27 individuals was approximately £380,000 in total or £14,000 per person. Following the introduction of the technology and sleep-in staff, this was reduced to £160,000 in total or £6000 per person.

Safety and quality

An audit was completed within the evaluation in which care staff were asked to rate the impact of the changes for the individuals within the service. This audit identified that there had been no increase in the number of night seizures, that incontinence pads had been effective for approximately two-thirds of the individuals who wore them and that all of their sleep patterns were either the same or improved. Independence had increased for 23 per cent of the individuals and privacy and autonomy had improved for 27 per cent. Approximately 35 per cent of staff reported that they were more trusting of the individuals' abilities, and there were no instances in which attempts to be more trusting had failed.

CHALLENGES IN IMPLEMENTING ASSISTIVE TECHNOLOGY

Choice Support found that the equipment was not always reliable, in particular the sensitivity of sensors and audibility of alarms. Incontinence pads were removed by some individuals and were not always sufficiently absorbent. Whilst many staff were supportive of the changes, managers reported that some were resistant, and the evaluation recommends that in the future such initiatives should provide more thorough training to equip staff members to more effectively use the technology and to demonstrate to them how it could have a positive impact. Sharing the benefits that have been realised for individuals in the service would also support the case for change.

What Real Life Options tried and learned

> ## Glynis' story
>
> Twelve people with a diverse range of support needs live in Stacey Drive. The home is built in the form of three bungalows linked together by a series of corridors. A number of people who live at Stacey Drive are now becoming elderly and frail, with their support needs increasing as a result. In the past, support staff used to check on all residents every hour, which was

disruptive for the residents. It also required a high staffing complement, as two waking-night staff were required to provide this level of monitoring.

Glynis lives at Stacey Drive, and during her person-centred review it was identified that she was not sleeping well at night. In fact, it was discovered that she was often getting up and walking about the property during the night. Of course, this disturbed Glynis' sleep and had a negative impact on her general well-being. Her intermittent sleep patterns were also disruptive for other residents.

Prior to the Transformation of Residential Care Homes (TORCH) programme, Real Life Options had worked with Tunstall regarding the use of telecare within residential care homes. Whilst these projects had some benefits, they had not worked as successfully as had been hoped, and the TORCH programme was therefore an opportunity to apply and build upon the learning from the previous projects at a larger scale. Tunstall became a member of the core group so that they could understand the overall change approach and inform its development. For Tunstall, the TORCH programme provided a means to think how their technology could be applied in tandem with person-centred practices, and linked to Just Enough Support, and thereby to think creatively how telecare could be used to improve the quality of life of people living in care homes while maintaining safety.

INTRODUCING THE TECHNOLOGY

Engineers from Tunstall visited all of the care homes and installed the infrastructure that would be required to enable the various sensors to be deployed. The main way that assistive technology was to be introduced was through the Just Enough Support sessions (see Chapter 3) so that they could learn about what each person required and suggest ways in which telecare could be of assistance.

Initially, Tunstall staff encountered that a number of Real Life Options staff were struggling with the idea of assistive technology, and even in some cases being negative about having it installed. They therefore raised this as something that was not working from their perspective at the monthly project group meeting. In the afternoon session, Tunstall representatives joined the mangers to work together to think about the possible root causes for the concerns of staff and to look at how these concerns could be addressed. The group looked at the challenges of embedding assistive technology and recognised that fundamentally this is a cultural change for staff. To successfully embrace it would require staff being able to see the benefits of assistive technology and the difference it could make, and where this fit within the Just Enough Support process.

Looking at the root causes of concerns about assistive technology, the group thought that one of them could be the belief that assistive technology is only for health and safety reasons, and typically might be used to reduce night-time support, which was a concern for staff. In order to start to address this, the group thought much more broadly around assistive technology and decided to conceptualise it from 'apps to assistive technology' (Figure 9.1). The group worked together to create a graphic looking at the different contributions that apps to assistive technology could make. This was framed around the 'Markers for Progress' that had been introduced by Think Local, Act Personal. To show how apps to assistive technology could be beneficial in terms of community, relationships, people doing the things that mattered to them, as well as addressing health and safety, each small group came up with different ideas for apps to assistive technology that they knew could help with those key areas.

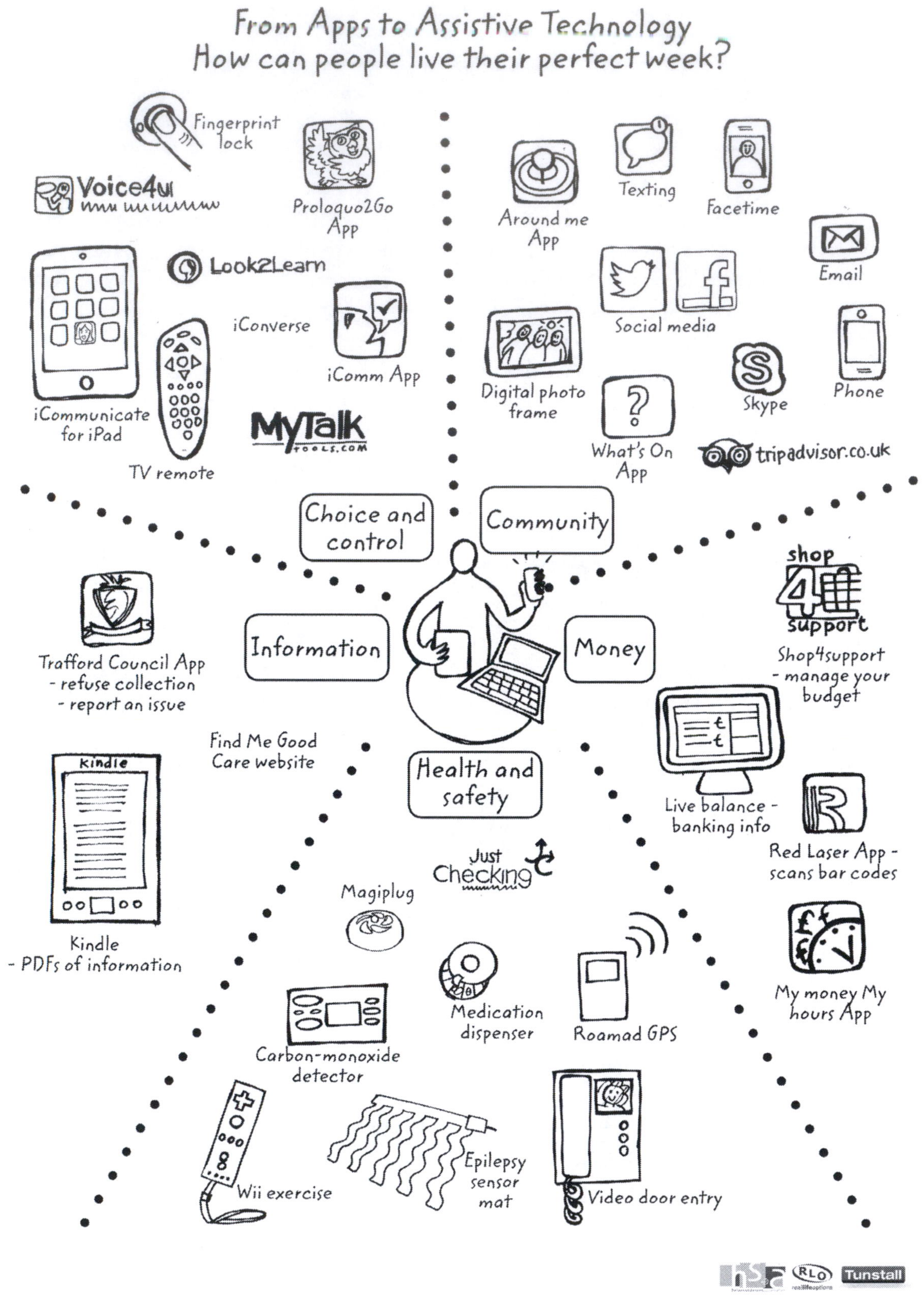

Figure 9.1 From apps to assistive technology[5]

---

5   The headings were adapted from the 'Markers for Progress' of Think Local, Act Personal (www.thinklocalactpersonal.org. uk), accessed 1 July 2014.

The first approach was to try to change staff and managers' understanding of the breadth of contribution that apps to assistive technology could make (Figures 9.2a and 9.2b). Next the group looked at how apps and assistive technology can increase and improve the quality of life for individuals across different areas, and not just around health and safety. To help staff understand this, the group created two scenarios, for two individuals, to both illustrate the process that starts at Just Enough Support through to person-centred review and how the decisions about assistive technology would be made, as well as how it would be implemented and reviewed. This created a very different process from the one that Tunstall was using at the time, and enabled Tunstall colleagues to co-create a much more person-centred approach to their installation of assistive technology.

Finally, the group looked at a different pathway for staff to learn about assistive technology (Figure 9.3). This started with supporting staff to think about the different ways they used apps and technology in different guises in their lives, to how they could understand specifically the benefit it could make for people they support and develop a specific pathway for staff to increase their understanding and appreciation of assistive technology.

The cultural and practical changes that introducing assistive technology requires was a journey on which the staff teams had started. These three approaches – thinking about the overall contribution of assistive technology to people's lives, the process for introducing assistive technology and a new learning pathway for staff – helped to pave the way. It was also recognised at this point that home managers were not always clear as to what the support needs were of each resident at night. Whilst it was thought that some residents were restless during the night and regularly left their bedroom, there was little evidence that this was actually the case. Real Life Options therefore asked Just Checking (Box 9.2) to work with them to understand the movement patterns of each of the residents. This information proved invaluable in identifying what staffing was actually required within each home at night and how assistive technology could be part of their support package.

Box 9.2 Overview of Just Checking

Just Checking is an assessment and care planning tool consisting of several movement and door contact sensors. These sensors are linked using passive infrared to a control box. This control box uses mobile signals to send data to a central system that can be accessed online using a secure login. The system updates every five minutes, meaning you get accurate and timely data which can pinpoint service user routines and possible issues within staff teams.[6]

6   See www.justchecking.co.uk for more information.

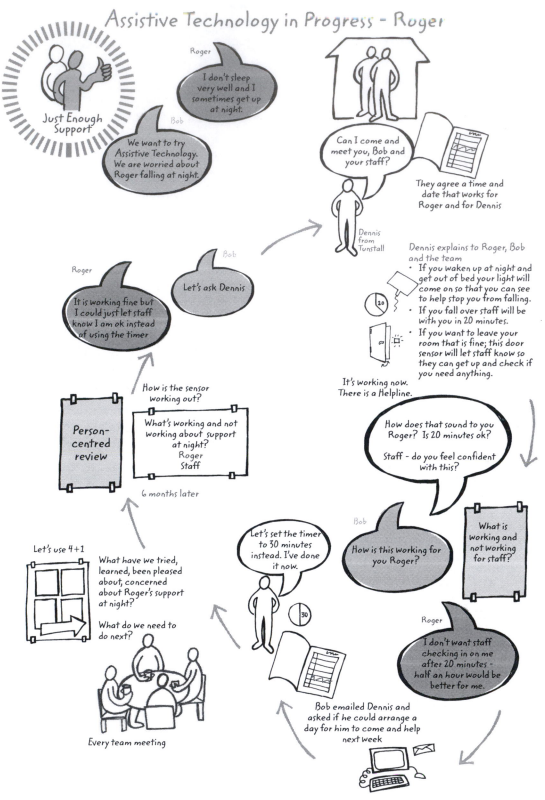

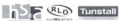

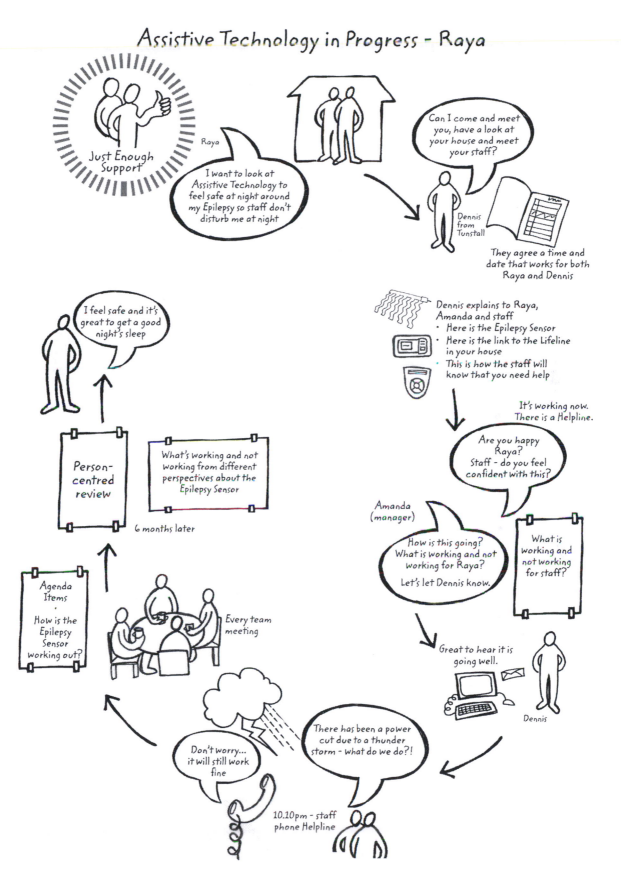

Figures 9.2a and 9.2b Assistive technology scenarios

From Apps to Assistive Technology Pathway

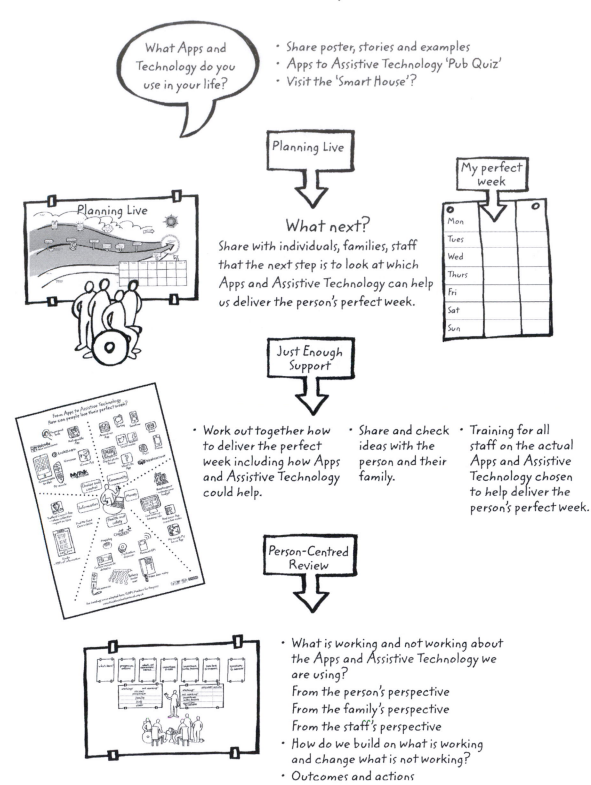

What Apps and Technology do you use in your life?

- Share poster, stories and examples
- Apps to Assistive Technology 'Pub Quiz'
- Visit the 'Smart House'?

Planning Live

Planning Live

My perfect week

Mon		
Tues		
Wed		
Thurs		
Fri		
Sat		
Sun		

What next?

Share with individuals, families, staff that the next step is to look at which Apps and Assistive Technology can help us deliver the person's perfect week.

Just Enough Support

- Work out together how to deliver the perfect week including how Apps and Assistive Technology could help.

- Share and check ideas with the person and their family.

- Training for all staff on the actual Apps and Assistive Technology chosen to help deliver the person's perfect week.

Person-Centred Review

- What is working and not working about the Apps and Assistive Technology we are using?
  From the person's perspective
  From the family's perspective
  From the staff's perspective
- How do we build on what is working and change what is not working?
- Outcomes and actions

Figure 9.3 Assistive technology learning pathway

IMPACT OF ASSISTIVE TECHNOLOGY

Glynis' story: Impact of assistive technology

The care and support that Real Life Options delivers at Stacey Drive has changed considerably since assistive technology was installed. The CareAssist portable alarm enables staff to receive alerts and respond as required rather than disturbing them every hour during the night. Furthermore, the alerts from the three bungalows are combined so that they can be picked up by a single CareAssist handset. This means that one member of staff can be available during the night to cover everyone. This saves resources, benefits everyone's daily life and creates a more settled environment that means everyone can sleep more soundly. It also frees up a staff member for day times so that residents can use their support time to do more things that they enjoy when they are awake during the day, which in turn can improve quality of life.

An enuresis sensor was installed on Glynis' bed and a sensor placed on her bedroom door. Staff are now able to target the care and support that she receives much more effectively, and she can therefore sleep more peacefully. Staff are alerted to any incidents that require support rather than having to check on Glynis every hour and further disturb her sleep and privacy.

The evaluation of the TORCH programme is not due to be completed until summer 2014, and the impacts of the assistive technology will therefore not be fully understood until that time. In the meantime, as the story of Glynis highlights, there is evidence that the technology is making some difference through enabling Real Life Options to better understand the needs of residents and develop the support accordingly.

CHALLENGES IN IMPLEMENTING ASSISTIVE TECHNOLOGY

Similar to Choice Support, there have been some problems with the technology. For example, the enuresis sensors can react at times due to sweat from the resident rather than an episode of incontinence, and the fall detectors sometimes indicate that someone has fallen when they have actually bent over. Some residents are also learning that if they stand up at night, a member of staff will come to their room even if they are not actually at risk. Not all homes and residents benefit as much as others from the technology due to their differing needs. Finally, whilst Tunstall is aware (and indeed is developing) the latest telecare equipment, the company is not yet informed of all of the possible types of assistive technology that are available, and this makes it difficult for Tunstall to recommend all potential equipment that could be of benefit.

Choice Support and Real Life Options have taken different approaches to the introduction of assistive technology and have found that there are complications regarding the functioning of the equipment and with staff and the people concerned engaging with it; however, both demonstrate that assistive technology can support the implementation of ISFs, and how important it is to support staff in exploring and understanding the benefits of assistive technology and see it as part of the ISF process (for example, as part of Just Enough Support).

Conclusion

RLO and Choice Support explored assistive technology alongside ISFs to further add to people's quality of life and to ensure that the funding available to them was used as efficiently as possible. They had different approaches to the introduction of the technology, but in both cases they identified that it was important to start with the support needs and aspirations of the individual.

They also learned that many care staff initially have concerns about such technology as they are concerned that it may lead to people accessing the service being at risk and a reduction in their hours of work. By listening and responding positively to staff's concerns it has been possible to introduce assistive technology. This has had positive benefits for some people, but there is potential for further improvements in the technology itself to ensure that it can work for more people. The services in which RLO and Choice Support introduced assistive technology support people with a learning disability. In Chapter 10 we learn about the different issues that may be connected with introducing ISFs with people who use mental health services.

Chapter 10

ISFs in Mental Health Services

Introduction

Most organisations that have introduced ISFs have done so within services for people with a learning disability. In this chapter we explore how these approaches can be transferred to services which support people with mental health problems. Mental health services are largely commissioned and provided by health services rather than social care services. The proportion of public funding that is used to support long-term residential care and supported living placements is less than that in learning disability, care management is not as engrained and policy is led by health organisations rather than social care bodies. These elements commonly result in commissioners and care managers in mental health services not being as familiar with individual funding models as those working in services for people with a disability. Furthermore, in mental health services it is often argued that the engagement of strong health disciplines (e.g. those of doctors, nurses and psychologists), combined with concerns regarding risk to self or others, have led to professional expertise and opinion being given a higher precedent over the views of people accessing services.

When Certitude and Look Ahead started to introduce ISFs within services for people with mental health problems, both organisations encountered a number of issues that were either particular or more pronounced than those within services for people with a learning disability. In this chapter we examine the specific challenges that they experienced and how these challenges have been overcome in order to make ISFs available to people with mental health problems.

Certitude: ISFs in residential care homes for people with mental health problems

Certitude initially sought to introduce ISFs within two residential care homes for people with mental health problems. This includes the home in which Jenny (who we met in Chapter 3) lives. The quality of life that Jenny was experiencing prior to the introduction of ISFs is highlighted below.

Jenny's story: Quality of life prior to ISFs

When staff first started to support Jenny, they noticed that her mental health was being affected by her preoccupation with rolling news and the impact of natural disasters, particularly hurricanes, tsunamis and earthquakes. Jenny was spending time alone in her room watching the news and working herself up to a state of complete fear and anxiety. Her many other fears, which included buses, trains, people from different countries and cultures, trees, planes, shops and crowds, were also restricting her opportunities to live a full life.

Certitude followed the processes outlined in Section 2; however, as these processes were principally developed within learning disability services, Certitude encountered a number of issues when they applied them in mental health. These issues are summarised below:

- Lack of familiarity with the language and principles of personalisation.

Whilst the principles are similar, the 'language' of personalisation, which is commonly used in relation to ISFs, was unfamiliar to staff working within mental health services. Staff members were much more at ease with terms related to 'recovery' and 'well-being'. Linked to this, person-centred practices seek to increase the choice for people accessing services about what they do and how they do it. This involves supporting them to have as much autonomy as possible in relation to balancing the potential risks with the potential benefits and developing their own sense of what is an 'acceptable' level of risk. In the words of the service manager, they were seeking to 'maximise risk but minimise danger'. Certitude found that community mental health professionals were more familiar with focusing on assessing risk to self and others and how to minimise it.

- People who used services did not believe they could have greater control.

Introducing 'personalisation' also required persuading people with mental health problems that they could make choices and do something different. Many people were not confident in their ability to do so and had internalised the importance of professional rather than personal perspectives. This meant that they needed ongoing support to believe that they had the right to make decisions about their care, and the confidence to communicate their views to staff.

- There was little individual funding available.

Applying the Care Funding Calculator within mental health services, it became clear that individuals were largely using their funding in relation to 'core' tasks delivered within the care homes and there was limited funding that was available to fund activities related to developing a broader quality of life. Furthermore, there was considerable variation in the support that individuals received with a few people requiring large amounts of support whilst others received relatively little.

- Addressing the issues within mental health services.

To address these particular issues, a number of additional initiatives were implemented within the mental health services. These issues included:

  ◦ New person-centred tools, including 'decision-making agreements', have been used to 'make personalisation practical' within mental health services.

  ◦ Support plans are now written from the perspective of the individual; for example, 'Paul wishes to be woken up at 9 a.m.' rather than 'wake Paul up at 9 a.m.'.

  ◦ Care staff have been encouraged to undertake shifts in other care homes to enable them to be comfortable in working with other individuals, and so that individuals become familiar with a wider range of staff who they may then ask to support them in relation to a particular activity.

  ◦ Recruitment of 'choice workers' who are not part of core staffing establishments and can be brought in to provide creative individual support.

  ◦ Rather than moving to a full ISF, each individual receives four hours of support each week that they can direct, with the opportunity to 'bank' these hours during a period of illness or to enable the resident to undertake a more time-consuming activity.

IMPACT OF CHANGES

Being clear about the number of hours of support that each individual has the flexibility to direct means that the person and their staff team are able to understand what is feasible within these resources. This has encouraged them to think about other personal and community resources that could be used, whereas in the past there was a general belief that public-sector funding should meet all of people's needs. The ISF process has also led to an improvement in care planning processes within the home, and this was highlighted by a Care Quality Commission inspection (Box 10.1).

> ## Box 10.1 Summary of Care Quality Commission inspection (January 2013)
>
> The home focuses on promoting the independence of the people who use the service, and this was evidenced through the activities on offer, the emphasis on daily living skills and the delivery of person-centred care.
>
> People's needs were assessed and care and treatment was planned and delivered in line with their individual care plan. People's care plans included tools used to provide individualised care planning. For example, 'people in my life' and 'places I go' tools were used to understand more about the person's behaviours and interests. In addition, the service used a local NHS Mental Health Trust's Recovery and Support Plan document to outline people's personal goals and how staff could support them to achieve those goals. People we spoke with outlined how the staff continued to involve them in the planning and delivery of their care. One person said, 'I meet with my key worker every four to six weeks to review the actions from my recovery star'. Another person told us, 'I discuss my progress with my key worker weekly'.

The impacts of introducing an ISF are best understood through considering the influence on individuals such as Jenny. She continues to suffer from a severe mental illness, and her condition continues to restrict her progress to some extent. For example, her relationship circle is limited by her reluctance to meet new people, and her negative outlook restricts her from recognising the positive changes she has made; however, her friends, family and the community mental health team who support her have seen a very positive improvement in her quality of life and the role she plays in determining how her life will be lived. After spending nearly 20 years in institutionalised settings, Jenny can now make more of her own choices, and the staff hope this will change the course of her life (see Jenny's story below).

Jenny's story continued: Changes for Jenny

With a greater understanding of her point of view, staff have been able to help Jenny take an interest in her appearance, and her self-esteem has risen. Now she regularly washes her hair, has purchased a hair dryer and visits the hairdresser. Staff have encouraged and supported her to have her teeth fixed and a front dental plate has changed her whole appearance. Her clothes are laundered every week and she changes her clothes daily.

The Certitude team also spends a lot of time talking to Jenny about what is happening on the news, and what is real and what is not real. Jenny has a great sense of humour and everyone has found that making her laugh can stop the spiralling fear and anxiety; however, only the staff she really connects with can usually do this.

Reflecting on the staff's experiences of supporting Jenny, Shaun Lindley, the manager of the home, has identified the practices below as being of particular importance to improving her quality of life and overall recovery through the ISF process.

People matching

Finding people that Jenny really likes to spend time with has had a particularly positive impact. Through 'people matching' (person-centred thinking tool: matching support) Jenny has been able to make it very clear that she prefers to be supported by people that she trusts and likes. The team respects these views and now Jenny is largely supported by the three of four members of staff she has indicated. She has given different reasons for each person and, for example, enjoys spending time with the manager because 'he's honest, tells it like it is, is funny and kind'.

Similarly, identifying Jenny's four 'personal control hours' per week has been significant. This is the time when Jenny chooses the activity she wishes to do, who supports her in doing it and when this takes place. As a result, she seems much happier to go out and take on activities which she had previously refused to do.

Choosing where to go and with whom

In the past, Jenny could name only about six places she was prepared to visit, and now her 'places map' has doubled. She used to refer to food shopping as a 'nightmare' but now takes the opportunity to visit a different supermarket every week, because she enjoys going out with the staff member who supports her. As she feels so at ease with him, she can be persuaded to try new and different shops. Furthermore, Jenny's newfound courage to explore has not stopped at shopping trips. Since she has been given the chance to choose which members of staff support her, she has taken a boat trip on the Thames, visited the Natural History Museum and the Southbank, and taken a day trip to the seaside and numerous outings to the cinema. She regularly enjoys walks in the park and trips to cafés, and she is rebuilding relationships with her family, that is, visiting her sister in Sutton and other relatives in Clacton. Choosing when she goes shopping and with whom has been key to the growth in Jenny's places map.

Making her own decisions

Jenny's decision-making agreement covered all the areas she wanted, including friendships, money, where she lives, holidays, medication, cleaning, cooking, laundry, work, benefits, family, personal care, food and nutrition, and shopping. This agreement certainly seems to have enabled her to express her views openly and honestly.

In all areas of her life Jenny has stated clearly what help she wants and how she wants that help delivered. For example, in relation to her not cooking, eating or drinking regularly, she has asked for staff to 'keep encouraging me to eat and drink', 'support me to cook, or if I'm not able, to cook for me', 'support me to shop' and 'encourage me to drink plenty of liquids and buy them for me'. Many of the choices and agreements born out of the decision-making agreement have been fed into Jenny's recovery-star action plan.

Look Ahead: ISFs in supported living for people with mental health problems

Look Ahead first introduced ISFs within their Coventry Road supported housing service, and then built on the learning from this project when they developed their rehabilitation service.

COVENTRY ROAD

Coventry Road, built and run by Look Ahead, is an accommodation-based supporting housing service for people with mental health problems. The service contains 20 self-contained flats and the support is purchased by the London Borough of Tower Hamlets. People who access the service are referred by the community mental health teams and often have a range of additional complex needs including offending behaviour, addiction to gambling and misusing substances. During the trial, the funding within the service was split between 'core' and 'flexi' (see Chapter 2). The individuals living at Coventry Road created their own personalised plans detailing how they wanted to change their lives and how they would use the flexible support hours and cash to do so. The plans were signed off jointly by the manager and the Look Ahead transformation lead officer.

The pilot at Coventry Road identified a number of improvements in the processes within the service and positive outcomes for the tenants in relation to their quality of life and their experience of receiving support (Table 10.1).

Table 10.1 *Positive impacts in pilot*

Type of impact	Before pilot	During pilot
Process	Tenants had little direct control over the staffing or other resources	Tenants had control over cash allocation and personalised support hours
	There was little opportunity to change staffing rota once this was in place (up to six weeks in advance)	Personalised support hours were adapted by request of the tenant
	There were lower staffing levels at weekends and evenings	Tenants often wanted to go out at weekends, and staffing levels were adapted as required
Quality of life	There were opportunities to access individual activities, but these activities were often promoted by staff	Tenants accessed a greater and more individualised range of activities
		There was improved self-image and confidence
		There was greater and better quality of contact with families
Experience of accessing service	Much staff time was taken encouraging tenants to engage with provided activities	Tenants had greater choice over activities and therefore needed less convincing
	Tenants often had low ownership of their support plans, despite person-centred principles being applied	Person-centred planning and control over the flexi resources resulted in greater tenant ownership
	25 per cent of tenants reported significant involvement in decision-making	70 per cent of tenants reported significant involvement

The pilot raised a number of important issues related to the introduction of ISFs within mental health services, as explained below.

Preparation

This is a significant change, and it is therefore vital to plan carefully what and who will be involved. Involving tenants at the planning stage both improves the model and enables them to become familiar with the opportunities that will be available to them. Linked to this, individuals and their staff will need support in thinking through the degree and type of choice that they had previously in order to understand what support would be required to successfully move to the new model. Look Ahead carried out one-to-one interviews with all the individuals in the service and staff. Researching and adapting existing resources and guidance can help to speed up the rate of improvement.

Workforce

Training and development can assist staff in understanding what will be required of them and sharing their concerns about their new responsibilities and connected skills. This applies to central support staff as well as direct care staff and their line managers. Moving to more individualised staffing rotas may lead to changes in working patterns, and in some circumstances staff members may not be guaranteed the same hours each week if tenants choose to spend their ISF differently or want to be supported by other staff members. Such changes may require consultation with the staff team regarding their terms and conditions.

Commissioners

Openness and trust in the relationship between the purchaser and providers is vital, as there are likely to be unfamiliar dilemmas to be addressed, for instance, if the tenant decided to buy something that would not usually come under the remit of health and social care services. Having a shared understanding of the purpose of the changes is also important so that both parties can be confident that their individual organisational aims will be met. A key issue in this regard is the potential for individuals to save up underspends in their cash or support hour allocations. Commissioners may also need to adapt their approach to gathering data for their needs analysis, as there will be additional and more individualised intelligence upon which to draw.

Individuals

Similar to the experience of Certitude, Look Ahead found that many of the individuals lacked confidence in their ability to make decisions about their mental health problems and how this had led them to be treated by society. They therefore required considerable support and encouragement to take greater control of their lives. This encouraged many of them to go beyond their 'comfort zones' to tell staff what they wanted (and who they wanted to support them), and to be able to change their minds even if this could be seen as inconveniencing staff. A key element of this process was adapting existing relationships and developing new relationships within their staff team, and both of these changes took time to become established.

Rehabilitation service

ISFs in the form of a flexi-cash allocation were built into the budget of the rehabilitation service as a key component of its recovery model. Many of the individuals group together for spending and this has led to informal peer support and improved social networks. Individuals accessing the service find that the trust given to them is very confidence building, motivating and inspires them to trust themselves to take positive steps in their recovery. The individual allocations also encourage people to think about and articulate their aspirations for the future, sometimes for the first time in years (Box 10.3). The potential for 'drift' has been recognised, though, in relation to individuals spending their ISFs on the basis of what they would like without considering how this would support their recovery.

Leroy's story: ISFs in rehabilitation services

Leroy's personal goals were to manage his own mental health, learn English, improve self-esteem and confidence, and live independently. Examples of his spend include getting a treadmill and bicycle to improve health and well-being, boat trips on the Thames, treating family to a meal at a restaurant, bowling, ice skating, London Zoo, circus, go-karting and tennis at the Paralympics. This was alongside other support to use local shops and facilities, GP registration, appointments with dentist and optician, and support around managing medication and medication routine which suited them, English language lessons.

Leroy did not have a hospital admission the whole time he was living at the rehabilitation service, despite a history of admissions. He moved into independent accommodation and is doing well.

In addition to the learning from the Coventry Road pilot, the following points have also been recognised as important components within the process of mental health services:

- Presenting the individual allocation as a tool for choice and control, and central to recovery, is a useful way to engage in the principles that lie behind ISFs.

- Having robust risk management and accountability processes are crucial for securing the support of commissioning and clinical partners.

- Building the individual allocation and actual spend into CPA reviews, meetings with care coordinators and team meetings ensures that the ISF becomes incorporated into day-to-day practice.

- Reviewing the spend quickly after the process begins enables individuals to relate progression to their increased choice and control, and shows that any successes can be developed further.

Conclusion

ISFs have been less commonly introduced in services for people with mental health problems than within services for people with a learning disability. In part this is due to their being more services for people with a learning disability that are block funded, but it is also connected with the professional language, culture and expectations within mental health services. Certitude and Look Ahead were not able to include all of the person's entitlement within their ISFs, but were able to identify an element of their support hours and/or budget that the person could have more control. From their experience, this and the person-centred practices introduced alongside ISFs, has led to a change in the dynamic between the person receiving support and their staff.

For a number of people this had made significant difference to their confidence in making decisions over their lives and in particular how they are supported. Certitude and Look Ahead have therefore been able to demonstrate that it is possible to introduce ISFs within mental health services. In Chapter 11 we find out about the experiences of Borough Care Ltd in relation to services for older people

ISFs in Older People's Services

Introduction

Bruce Lodge is home to 43 people living with dementia in Offerton, Stockport. People from Borough Care Ltd and the manager of Bruce Lodge, Lisa Martin, were supported by a joint leadership to implement the principles of ISFs. This chapter describes how the leadership team worked together to define success and learn what was happening before introducing ISFs, and how Lisa and her team introduced one-page profile meetings, individual time, learning logs and person-centred reviews. Bruce Lodge was the first place to introduce the foundations of ISFs to people living with dementia, and this chapter describes some of the impact of this on the people, families, staff and the organisation.

The leadership team

The leadership team was made up of people from Borough Care Ltd (CEO and deputy), Bruce Lodge (Lisa, her deputy and seniors at various meetings) and Stockport Council (commissioners, heads of workforce, department of quality and contracts). The purpose of the leadership team was to implement personalisation and the principles of ISFs in a way that did not cost the commissioners or the provider more money (i.e. within existing resources). The only additional resource was the commissioner buying in the support from a consultant to facilitate the process, and a trainer to provide direct support to Lisa and her colleagues; therefore, the leadership team had two related purposes for the project:

1. to implement individualised hours (the resource available to people as their ISF)

2. to deliver more personalised support on a day-to-day basis to each individual.

Before the project began, the leadership team completed three tasks: they organised for baseline data to be collected, defined what success would look like and developed an internal and external communications plan.

BASELINE DATA

The leadership team used three ways to gather baseline data. The first way was to use the care homes self-assessment 'Progress for Providers' to see how personalisation was being delivered. The other two ways were the Quality of Interactions Schedule, an observational audit tool, and completing a Dementia Care Map. (The before-and-after data are discussed in Chapter 12.)

DEFINING SUCCESS AND A COMMUNICATION PLAN

The leadership team developed a 'one-page strategy' to communicate what success looked like from different perspectives, how they planned to deliver this and how this would be measured. They thought that success for people living at Bruce Lodge would be for people to be able to say, 'I'm supported by people who know me, and they act on what matters to me now and on how I want to be supported'.

To deliver a truly personalised service, people need to be known and treated as individuals, in a way that reflects both what matters to them and how they want to be supported. This would be reflected in people's one-page profiles: 'I'm listened to and heard, and supported to make choices and decisions'.

The leadership team wanted people to be involved in their day-to-day life in a way that worked for them. They wanted people to be listened to and heard, and to make choices and decisions, as this reflects the key principles around personalisation. This would happen through people deciding how they wanted to use their individual time and in staff acting on the information in people's one-page profiles: 'I have individual time each month and choose what I do and who supports me'.

Because the team wanted to implement ISFs, they obviously needed a success statement that reflected this: people having individual time each month, and choosing what they do and who supported them, was fundamental to this. The leadership team also wanted the project to make a positive difference in the lives of staff. They wanted staff to feel listened to, and to be able to contribute to the lives of the people they supported – to the home and the success of the organisation overall. The leadership team wanted staff to feel that their hobbies and interests were matched to how people living at Bruce Lodge wanted to spend their individual time. In addition to this, they wanted staff to have an increased sense of job satisfaction from doing a great job and supporting people in a person-centred way on a day-to-day basis.

There are lots of initiatives and projects aspiring to change the lives of people with dementia. This project was underpinned by the belief that it is crucial to change the staff's experience as part of this. As well as defining success for people who live at Bruce Lodge, and staff, the leadership team looked at what success meant for both Borough Care Ltd and Stockport Council. Figure 11.1 shows the final version of the one-page strategy, with what success looked like, the person-centred practices that they would use to deliver this and how they would measure success. They suggested different names for the project, and the seniors made the final decision, calling it 'My Home, My Life, My Choice'.

The one-page strategy was a key part of the communication plan, which focused on internal and external stakeholders for both Borough Care Ltd and Stockport Council. It included information in newsletters, having the project as a standard agenda item at key meetings, workshops for other providers, briefings for elected members and video blogs for Stockport Council's intranet, as well as sharing through social media.

TRAINING AND COACHING

Once the leadership team had defined success, gathered baseline information and developed their communications plan, they developed a detailed project plan to implement the ISFs. The key elements of this plan were as follows:

- Identify the resource available.

- Develop one-page profiles with all staff.

- Facilitate 'one-page profile meetings' with individuals and their families.

- Implement 'individual time' on the rota and learning logs to record progress.

- Facilitate person-centred reviews every six months to review progress.

Figure 11.2 provides a summary of the process to implement an ISF for an individual who lives at Bruce Lodge.

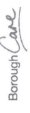

My Home, My Time, My Choice
Personalising Care Homes
One-Page Strategy

What success means from different perspectives

People living at Bruce Lodge
- I am involved in the day-to-day life of where I live in a way that makes sense to me
- I am supported by people who know me, and act on what matters to me now, for my future and how I want to be supported
- I am listened to and heard, and supported to make choices and decisions
- I have individual time each month and choose what I do and who supports me

Staff at Bruce Lodge
- Our hobbies and interests are matched to how people living at Bruce Lodge want to spend their individual time
- We are listened to and able to contribute to the lives of the people we support, the home and success of the organisation
- We get satisfaction from doing a great job and supporting people in a person-centred way on a day-to-day basis and with their individual hours

Borough Care
- We are delivering a person-centred service that people have confidence in, and want to buy
- We demonstrate and share good practice in delivering personalised services for people living with dementia in care homes
- We know and act on what's working and what's not working for people using and working in our services

Stockport Council
- We are commissioning personalised services which are safe and offer real choice for the people living with dementia in Stockport
- We are working in active partnership with providers to deliver personalised services for people living in care homes
- We share what we are learning locally, regionally and nationally

How we are delivering this

People living at Bruce Lodge
- One-page profiles
- Communication charts and decision making agreements
- Working/Not working
- Outcomes for individual time
- Learning logs (for individual time)
- Matching staff

Staff at Bruce Lodge
- Staff one-page profiles
- Matching staff
- Working/Not working

The Leadership Team Borough Care and Stockport Council with HSA
- Project team one-page profiles
- Working/Not working
- Doughnut – to clarify responsibilities in delivering this
- Communication chart – sharing learning locally, regionally and nationally

How we are measuring this

People living at Bruce Lodge
- Number of people with one-page profiles that meet standards, with Working/Not working
- Number of people with communication charts/decision making agreements
- Number of people who have clear specified outcome for using their 2 hours individual time
- Increase in scores from Dementia Care Map

Staff at Bruce Lodge
- Number of staff with one-page profiles that meet standards
- Matching staff used for each individual based on how they want to spend their individual 2 hours
- Percentage of Learning Logs used to capture learning from how people spent their individual time
- Increase in scores from Progress for Providers

The Leadership Team Borough Care and Stockport Council with HSA
- Percentage of people living at Bruce Lodge whose individual time is delivered by key worker. We are looking for staff to be chosen individually and not expecting this to always be the keyworker
- Analysis of how the 2 hours are used per person. We are expecting to see variety, for example, some people having their 2 hours a month in 4 half hour sessions
- Percentage of people who use their individual time outside of Bruce Lodge. We are looking for a high percentage of people to use their time to be in the community
- Range of creative options (versus traditional options) tried to enable people to use their 2 hours in the way that they want
- Increase in the scores from Dementia Mapping and Observation Schedule
- Increase in scores from Progress for Providers
- Percentage of actions achieved from Dementia Mapping recommendations
- Number of places/ways where information about this has been shared
  a) Internally
  b) externally (regionally and nationally)

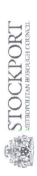

Figure 11.1 One-page strategy for My Home, My Life, My Choice

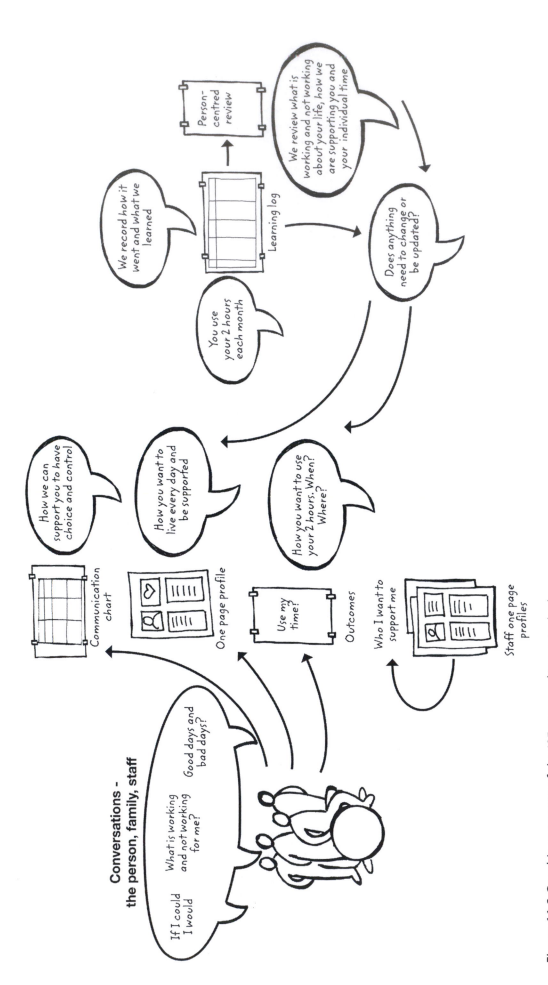

Figure 11.2 Graphic summary of the ISF process (Bruce Lodge)

Identifying the funding resource

The leadership team did not try to deconstruct the block contract into individual budget allocations. They knew that this would be important in the future but took the pragmatic decision to identify how many hours could be in each person's personal control in Bruce Lodge. Practically, the leadership team did not think that any less than two hours would be worth doing, and this led to agreeing on a 'budget' of two hours a month per person. This had to be found within the existing time that staff had, as there was no additional allocation of staff or money.

Developing one-page profiles with staff

Every staff member (including administrative staff, night staff and housekeeping staff) developed a one-page profile by taking part in a three-hour on-site training session. The three-hour session was repeated three times to enable all staff to attend. There were two reasons for starting with staff one-page profiles. The first reason was to enable Lisa to match staff to how people wanted to use their individual time on the basis of shared interests. (The staff member's interests and hobbies are recorded in a one-page profile.) The second reason was to be able to support staff in a more personalised way and for staff to be able to get to know each other more, as this staff member at Bruce Lodge relates:

> The one-page profile was introduced probably about ten months ago, and I have personally found it to be really good for us as staff. Some staff were transferred from different homes and have worked here for eight to ten years. We really didn't know much about some people, for example, we didn't know they have children, or that they like going out at weekends. It was really interesting to learn that people have a life outside of work.
>
> The one-page profiles told us the things we have in common, and then we were matched to people and them to us. We found we had more interesting things to talk about than we would have before.

One-page profile meetings with individuals and their families

Lisa and the trainer planned 90-minute informal meetings with each individual and their family over a period of four months. (The one-page profile meeting process is described in Chapter 2.) Each meeting resulted in:

- a detailed one-page profile that described what is important to the person and how they want to be supported

- the person's chosen 'outcome', that is, how they want to use their individual time.

Mary's story: One-page profile meeting

Gill, the trainer, describes the one-page profile meeting with Mary:

> Mary's one-page profile was developed from thinking with Mary, her daughter Brenda and Lisa about good days and bad days. We were able to capture into Mary's one-page profile these key things which must be present if life is to be as good as it possibly can be. They were better able to support Mary well by being clear that a bad day was caused by her missing out on fun things that were happening in the home due to the amount of physical support she needed, and as a result, staff were much more mindful of ensuring she didn't miss out because her one-page profile served as their day-to-day job description. It also meant that staff were able to have good conversations

with her by talking about things of interest to her, as described in her profile, such as Brenda, family life and the Royal family. Her favourite music can always be heard when she is on bed rest, and staff know to ensure her TV is on if any of her favourite programmes are on. If Mary says something that may be upsetting, everyone knows to respond with a soft approach and learn from watching staff who know her well. She swears at people, but her daughter asked that staff never be offended by that. It's not vulgar and not intended with any malice. So I recommend in such cases that staff have some banter with Mary, or let her know very softly that they feel upset at what she's said. She usually responds very well and will want to hold people's hand and let them know it was said in jest.

Looking at Mary's good days and bad days, and what is working and not working for her, provided rich, detailed information about what is important to her and gave clues about how she wants to be supported, and this tended to make her day-to-day experience how she wanted it to be. Asking different questions led to different conversations that led to a thorough understanding about what matters to Mary and how she wants to be supported. This is the information needed to ensure a person's support is tailored to their needs and aspirations, and that is the very bedrock of personalisation. Figure 11.3 shows Mary's one-page profile.

Implementing and learning from 'individual time'

Lisa used staff's one-page profiles to identify the best match between how the person wanted to use their individual time and a staff member who shared that particular hobby or interest. Sometimes there was only one obvious person, and where there were a couple of possibilities, the person themselves could choose and make the final decision. Once this decision was made, Lisa put this on the rota. Within two to three weeks after the meeting, the person started their 'individual time'.

The staff member was expected to take a photo and complete a 'learning log' after the individual time. The learning log was used to adjust what we were doing in supporting the person to make it work better (What did we learn about how best to support the person?), and to update the one-page profile as necessary (Have we learned anything more about what is important to the person and what we appreciate about them?).

Mary wanted to use her individual time outdoors in the park with fresh air on her face, feeding ducks and visiting cafés. Lisa matched her to Karen. Figure 11.4a shows an example learning log, and Figure 11.4b shows what was learned from it.

What is important to Mary

- Brenda, her daughter, who visits at least twice a week. Maureen, Mary's other daughter who lives in Harrogate and visits every few weeks. Michael, Anthony, Jay and Katy, Mary's grandchildren.
- Mary loves her food – fish and chips are her favourite.
- Chocolate is a must – Mary has a supply in her cupboard.
- To have her hair done each week.
- Mary loves hugs and affection.
- Listening to her selection of CDs which she keeps in her bedroom.
- Having a sing song is always good.
- Banter – having good rapport with those supporting her.
- Mary loves to go out in the fresh air.
- Fish and chips in Morrison's café is her favourite.
- Watching The Proms, anything to do with royalty – changing of the guard, Songs of Praise – hymns are favourites of Mary.
- That you chat to her lots – about Brenda, about your own families, what you have been doing. Mary will enjoy listening.
- Having small children around her.
- Lots of compliments are a must, Mary visibly grows.
- Her room – her pictures of her family, her CD player, her cushions and throws

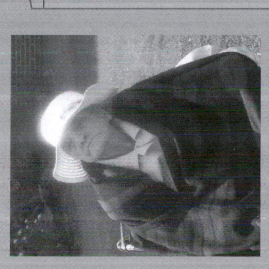

What those who know Mary best say they like and admire about her

Salt of the earth!
A great woman
A wonderful character
Her funny sayings
Says it as it is

How we can best support Mary

- Always be aware that due to the number of interventions (as detailed in the care plans around skin integrity) there is a real danger. Mary may miss out on the fun things that are going on – be mindful of this and ensure Mary is involved as far as is possible or that she wants to be.
- Know that Mary's head leans back and so she only drinks from a feeder cup or with a straw – see care plan for detail.
- Mary will swear – never be offended, it is not vulgar and isn't intended with any malice.
- Mary needs a supporter who will have banter and fun with her – who can pick out words Mary says to keep the conversation alive.
- You need to know Mary well to understand her – she will often not mean what she says – she may be unhappy with you and tell you straight, but learn from her family and the staff who know her best.
- Know that Mary uses a special shampoo that Brenda brings in – the hairdresser who washes Mary's hair each week is aware of this.
- Know that Mary responds well if she knows she has said something upsetting to you – it works best with a soft approach and learn from watching staff who know Mary well.
- Mary's chocolate is in the small cupboard in her room, ensure she is offered some each day!

Figure 11.3 Mary's one-page profile

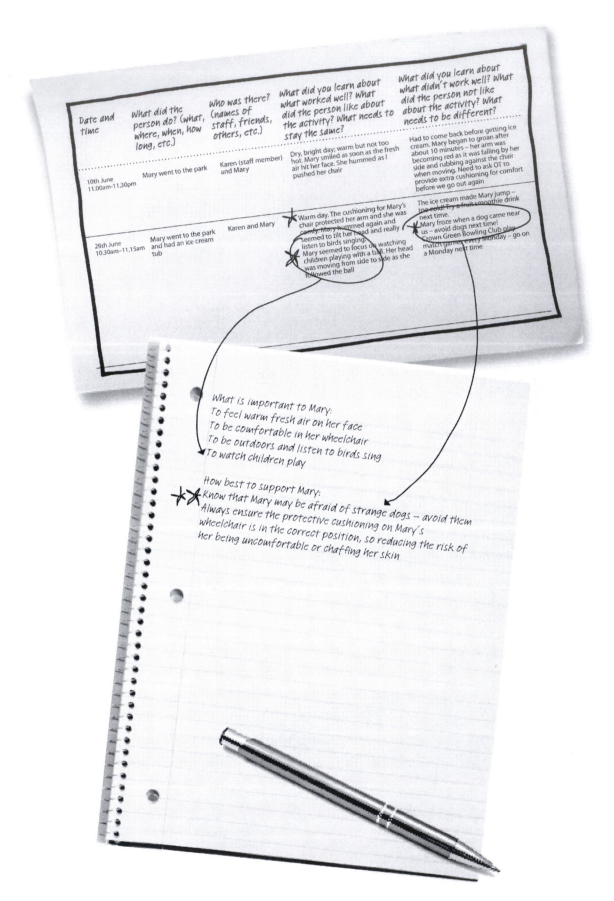

Figure 11.4 (a) A learning log for Mary's individual time and (b) what was learned from the log

Listening and reviewing progress

The leadership team met monthly to review progress. They had multiple ways of gathering feedback each month. This feedback included:

- comments on 'comments cards' from families and professionals

- what was working and not working from the staff's perspectives

- what was working and not working from the manager's perspective

- what was working and not working from the consultant's perspective

- a dashboard of metrics taken directly from the 'how we will know how we are doing' section of the one-page strategy.

At each meeting they would review all the comments, metrics and what was working and not working. They would then develop solutions and actions to change what was not working. This led directly to the following:

- developing a new group activities timetable taken directly from the information from people's one-page profiles

- developing night-time one-page profiles to enable night staff to deliver more personalised support

- creating a range of ways to support people to display the photographs of how they used their 'individual time'

- exploring what staff would like to do in the future and adding a second page to the staff one-page profiles: 'If I could, I would'

- developing a community map of where people were using their individual time

- a process for developing one-page profiles with volunteers and matching them to individuals

- specific efforts to engage with local faith communities

- exploring circles of support as a way to connect people with their communities.

After six months, individuals at Bruce Lodge started to have person-centred reviews to reflect again on what was working and not working for them (Figure 11.5), and whether they wanted to change how they were using their individual time.

At the end of 12 months, the leadership team used 'Working Together for Change' to aggregate learning and information from the first 12 people who had had a person-centred review. This meant that the future development of the project could be led by what people living with dementia identified as their priorities, based on what was working and not working from their perspective.

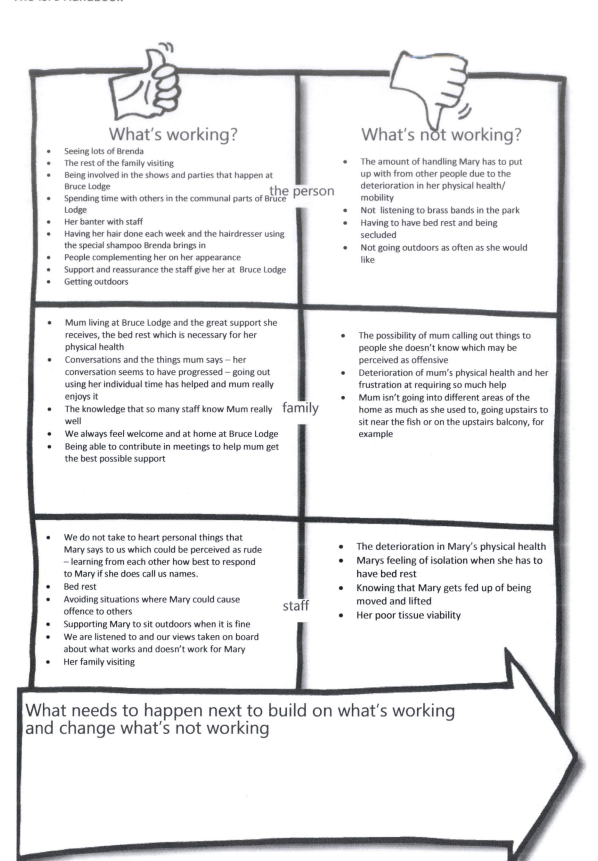

Figure 11.5 'Working and not working' for Mary, from different perspectives, from her person-centred review

What difference have ISFs made?

Real personalisation requires a cultural change from a task-focused ethos to one that values what matters most to the people being supported. Through implementing one-page profiles and individual time, this cultural change has started to take place at Bruce Lodge (Figure 11.6). Staff now naturally involve people in tasks and so living and working at Bruce Lodge becomes a shared experience. Staff no longer wear uniforms and there is little sense of a 'them and us' culture: people living at Bruce Lodge are respectfully perceived as being the experts in their own lives.

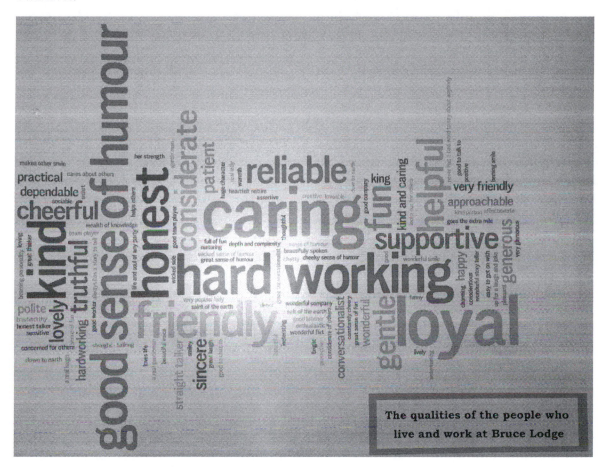

Figure 11.6 What people who live and work at Bruce Lodge appreciate about each other (taken from everyone's one-page profiles)

Lisa Martin, the manager, says the following about the benefits of the approaches used during this personalisation project:

> Matching individuals and staff around shared interests has been a real win-win situation: for the person, doing something that matters to them with someone who is enthusiastic about it; and for the staff, having an opportunity to share a hobby or interest at work.

Lisa describes how staff are going the extra mile in demonstrable ways, thinking about the people living at Bruce Lodge even when not at work. For example, the housekeeper Roy looked for some of his old classical CDs as he knew John who lived at Bruce Lodge also enjoyed that genre of music. Roy set John up with the CDs playing in a small lounge where he would not be disturbed and then went about his work, popping back in to see how John was enjoying the music now and again.

The benefits have been significant for individuals and their families too. Maureen, the daughter of Winifred (who lives in the home), states:

> Mum can be heard singing aloud as she carries out the chores she did so routinely in her own home before she moved here. She is happier, chatting more, using fuller sentences, is sleeping better and generally more alive.

Lynn, whose mother recently came to live at Bruce Lodge, commented, 'It was the idea that mum would be able to continue doing some of those things that brought her such joy, such as going to a show or to see horses, that made us choose Bruce Lodge'.

REALLY LISTENING

May, who is living with dementia, states:

> If people would ask me, I could still tell them what I want – I just need a bit more help getting those things these days. I can't just go and have a coffee in my favourite café because I may not find my way back. Life isn't worth living without those small joys, so what do we do?

May's comment is an example from the conversations that took place at the one-page profile meetings. The process meant that the person themselves and those who loved and cared most about the people living at Bruce Lodge were listened to well. Asking different questions led to different conversations that gave a thorough understanding of what was going to work for each individual. In turn, this made people think differently about how support was provided. This information ensured that each person's support was tailored to their needs and aspirations – the very bedrock of personalisation.

Overall, the project has made everyone involved feel a greater sense of connection to Bruce Lodge: staff, family members and volunteers are bringing in things to support other people's individual time.

WORKING AND LIVING TOGETHER

Team members say they feel they know each other much better as a result of developing one-page profiles. They have different conversations based on what they have learned about each other and therefore have become a closer team, and they are much clearer about what good support looks like to each other. Lisa also said she is much clearer about what good support looks like to individual staff members, and she has improved supervision sessions, team meetings and the way the team works together and with individuals as a result.

Choosing the right person to provide support during individual time was arguably one of the most important decisions that made a difference to people living at Bruce Lodge, as doing something we want to do can still be a miserable experience if we are not with someone we like. Using staff one-page profiles and those of people living at Bruce Lodge was key to ensuring people had the best possible experience during their individual time, because it meant they had a say in who they spent time with and who would provide their support. Staff are describing their approach as 'simply the way we work'.

The activity programme also looks totally different as each group activity is designed around the individuals taking part, reflecting on what is important to them and being led by a staff member who also has an interest in that activity. For example, groups now take part in baking sessions and Bible sessions.

Conclusion

Bruce Lodge's experience has been that ISFs can also lead to positive changes within older peoples' services. They have seen impacts for the people who live in the home, the staff and for the organisation. The people living in the home now receive more individualised support and a number have increased well-being as a result. Families have a greater sense of connection to Bruce Lodge and now bring in things to support other people's individual time. For staff there has been a change in culture from task focus to relationship focus, they are getting to know each other more and are willing to go the 'extra mile' in demonstrable ways. They increasingly see this as 'simply the way we work'.

Borough Care Ltd as an organisation have received over one hundred per cent increase in enquiries to Bruce Lodge with over 50 per cent of these specifically mentioning the 'personalised time'. There has also been a positive impact on their reputation within Stockport Council and nationally – for example they were finalists in National Dementia Awards in the innovation category.

Finally Joan, the commissioner of Borough Care Ltd, commented:

> Through the work at Bruce Lodge, Borough Care Ltd has demonstrated that ISFs can be also a powerful tool to facilitate changes in practice within residential care homes for older people living with dementia, despite the limited resources that are often available to such services. One of the reasons for their success was their determination to keep their focus on the differences that ISFs could make to the quality of life of people living in the home.

One of the key elements within the introduction of ISFs in Bruce Lodge was to measure the impacts. In Chapter 12 we learn about the approach taken by them and other organisations in relation to impact measurement.

Understanding the Impact

Introduction

Organisational change initiatives are generally introduced in response to an area of practice or business that is not going as well as hoped, or to take advantage of an opportunity for further growth or improvement. In both scenarios, it is common for organisations to be somewhat vague about what the overall purpose of the changes will be and even vaguer about what success will look like at the end of the project. This lack of clarity often becomes amplified over time as projects have to adapt to other challenges and opportunities that are encountered. They are also frequently not 'completed' as discrete projects and instead get subsumed into new initiatives. This means that it is possible for organisations to spend considerable time, energy and resources trying to change something without being sure about what has actually been achieved at the end of the process.

In care services, the most important impacts are, of course, those that affect the lives of people who are receiving support and their family carers. There are, though, other impacts in which organisations will be interested, including the well-being of their staff, the efficiency with which they use their resources and the degree to which they fulfil the expectations of their commissioners. In addition to assessing these impacts, organisations may also want to understand what has worked and what could be improved in the change process, and to identify other potential improvements in the service in question. Gathering, reflecting and acting on this variety of data can be a complex process, particularly if the people who access services have different communication methods or have limited understanding of their situation and support.

There is no one way to try to understand impact and change processes connected with the introduction of ISFs. The methods used by each organisation need to respond to the nature of the changes and the context in which they have been introduced. They are also influenced by the resources and time available, and if, for example, there is funding to bring in an external organisation, such as a university, to support with an evaluation.

This chapter highlights the different approaches used by three of our case study organisations – Choice Support, Bruce Lodge and Real Life Options – which are broadly grouped under the 'methods' that they adopted: surveys and audits, observational approaches and Working Together for Change (WTFC).

Surveys and audits

Choice Support commissioned Bucks New University to undertake an evaluation of their ISF programme. The first stage of this evaluation[1] was concerned with the changes to the night staffing. It began with Bucks New University trying to understand more about the change process through discussing what was planned with the services managers. This approach to an evaluation is often called 'theory based', in that the thinking behind why a change will work and what it will deliver is made clear at the beginning of the project (often called the 'programme theory'). During these initial discussions, Bucks New University was seeking to establish the following in particular:

---

1   Ellis, R. and Sines, D. (2012) *Better Nights: Evaluation of Choice Support in Southwark.* Sheffield: Choice Support.

- who the key stakeholders were (i.e. people and groups which would be affected by, or have a perspective on, the changes)

- what outcomes Choice Support was hoping to achieve

- how success could be identified and measured

- what change processes would be deployed.

Building on the information gathered from these discussions, an audit tool was developed to measure against two of the main outcomes: management of risk and improving the quality of life of the individuals accessing the services. This incorporated 27 aspects of the change process and the anticipated outcomes (e.g. see Box 12.1). The audit tool was completed by a support worker who knew the individual resident well, with the worker's assessment being confirmed by their manager. The evaluation team also wanted to gain the perspectives of the close family members and the wider support staff team regarding the impacts on the residents. They recognised that the full version of the audit would potentially be off-putting in length and require details of which these stakeholders might not be aware. Shorter audits were therefore developed for these stakeholder groups which asked about the impact on the overall quality of life and risk to the residents. These audits also explored the views of these stakeholders regarding the motivation and management of the change process, and for the staff, how the changes had affected their working lives.

Box 12.1 Examples of aspects included in audit tool

Night seizures:

- The service user does not suffer night seizures.

- The service user has suffered night seizures more frequently than previously.

- The service user has suffered night seizures less frequently than previously.

- The service user has suffered night seizures at the same rate as previously.

Consistency of support:

- The new shifts have led to a deterioration in consistency of support for this service user.

- The new shifts have had no impact on consistency of support for this service user.

- The new shifts have improved the consistency of support for this service user.

This audit process provided valuable information regarding the impact of the programme and the process of change. The evaluation report noted, though, that there were difficulties in identifying family members with sufficient contact with the residents to complete the audits, and that ideally the person themselves should rate any impacts on their care or their quality of life. This highlights that understanding the impact of ISFs is a complex task and one that is generally limited by available time and resources; however, being clear about why a particular methodology has been chosen, and its strengths and weaknesses, helps to put the results in context and ensure that any conclusions have greater validity.

To understand the impact of the Transformation of Residential Care Homes (TORCH) programme, Real Life Options piloted a provider version of the Personalisation Outcomes Evaluation Tool (POET). This was developed by In Control and the Centre for Disability Research at Lancaster University to provide a standard approach to measuring the impact that personal budgets are having on people's lives. POET has been used within two national surveys in England as well as by local authorities and in relation to personal health budgets. It therefore has a proven track record of capturing the outcomes that people have achieved with such budgets, which can be helpful in comparing the impact of a project with other such initiatives. POET involves people who hold the budget or a trusted other person rating their quality of life in relation to a number of key aspects (Table 12.1). These data are completed online with each person having an anonymised reference number, with the website providing a range of analyses through a simple process.

Generally, the person who receives the personal budget completes POET because it is difficult to comment on someone else's quality of life, as we all see different elements as being more important; however, the people involved in the TORCH programme were not able to complete such forms by themselves, and these people were therefore led by the services managers. Due to time pressures, the POETs were largely completed by the manager building on existing information. (In the future they will be completed within the person's person-centred review with all those present contributing to the final rating of each quality of life.) The people who have contributed to the ratings are also recorded so that it is clear whose perspectives have been gathered. The managers of Real Life Options complete the POET for people before those people participate in the Planning Live process and then repeat the POET six months afterwards.

The provider version of POET being trialled with Real Life Options also asks about the stage of the ISF process that the person has reached and the degree to which they have achieved (or not) their three most important goals. The helps and hindrances related to these goals are also gathered. This helps Real Life Options to understand the differences that the TORCH project has made, and other changes that have impacted on these differences.[2]

Table 12.1 *Example of aspects of quality of life within Personalisation Outcomes Evaluation Tool*

Aspect of quality of life	Very good	Good	Fair	Poor	Very poor
Leisure (enjoys hobbies and recreational activity)					
Communication (with people around them)					
Relationships between the person and their support staff					

---

2   See www.in-control.org.uk/what-we-do/poet-%C2%A9-personal-outcomes-evaluation-tool.aspx.

Bruce Lodge and Real Life Options used the Progress for Providers self-assessment tool to understand how their practice had developed during their change programmes. Progress for Providers is a self-assessment tool to enable providers to check how they are doing in delivering personalised services. It focuses on three dimensions of practice: that related to the individual, that related to families and that related to staff (see Boxes 12.2–12.4). Managers rate themselves and their service on each of the statements below on a scale between 1 and 5:

- Levels 1 and 2 signify that residential homes are beginning to look at and address personalisation.

- Levels 3 and 4 signify that residential homes are delivering person-centred care.

- Level 5 signifies excellence, that the home is delivering personalised support, including individualised funding.

If completed on a periodic basis, Progress for Providers provides insights into how managers' use of the person-centred practices that underpin the successful deployment of ISFs has changed over time.

Box 12.2 Progress for Providers: Section 1 – The Person

1. We see and treat the person as an individual, with dignity and respect.

2. We understand the person's history.

3. We know and act on what matters to the person.

4. We know and act on what the person wants in the future (outcomes).

5. We know and respond to how the person communicates.

6. The person is supported to make choices and decisions every day.

7. We know exactly how the person wants to be supported and how to support them to be fully part of everyday life.

8. We know what is working and not working for the person, and we are changing what is not working.

9. We support people to initiate and maintain friendships and relationships.

10. We support the person to be part of their community and civic life.

11. The environment is pleasant, homely and busy.

12. We support individuals to be in the best possible physical health.

13. There is a person-centred culture of respect and warmth.

14. People have personal possessions.

15. Meal times are pleasurable, flexible, social occasions.

Box 12.3 Progress for Providers: Section 2 – The Family

1. The home is a welcoming place for families.

2. Family members have good information.

3. Families contribute their knowledge and expertise.

4. We support family relationships to continue and develop.

Box 12.4 Progress for Providers: Section 3 – The Staff and Manager

1. We have knowledge, skills and understanding of person-centred practices.

2. Staff are supported individually to develop their skills in using person-centred practices.

3. Our team has a clear purpose.

4. We have an agreed way of working that reflects our values.

5. Staff know what is important to each other and how to support each other.

6. Staff know what is expected of them.

7. Staff feel that their opinions matter.

8. Staff are thoughtfully matched to people, and rotas are personalised to people who are supported.

9. Recruitment and selection is person centred.

10. We have a positive, enabling approach to risk.

11. Training and development is matched to staff.

12. Supervision is person centred.

13. Staff have appraisals and individual development plans.

14. Meetings are positive and productive.

Figure 12.1 demonstrates the increase of scoring via Progress for Providers for Bruce Lodge. This was initially completed in April 2012 and reviewed in August 2013. This information can be used to facilitate discussions regarding the areas of practice in which progress has been made and identify those areas that need further work.

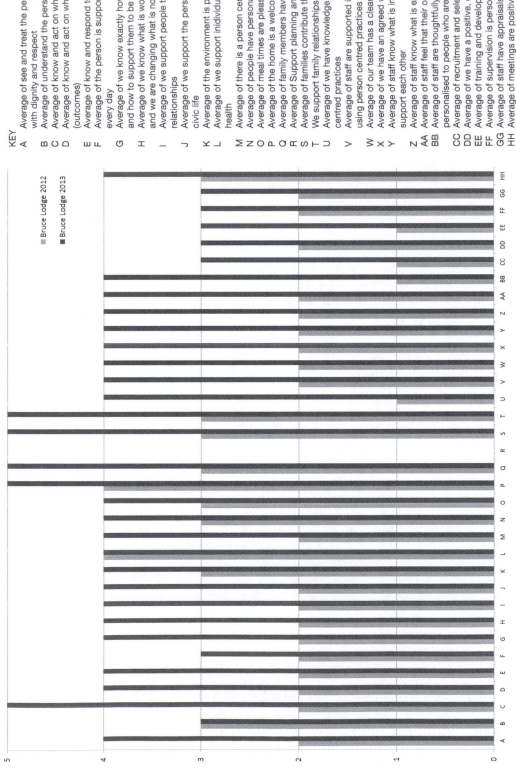

Figure 12.1 The increase of scoring via Progress for Providers for Bruce Lodge
Dark grey bars refer to April 2012, and light grey bars refer to August 2013

Bruce Lodge 2012
Bruce Lodge 2013

OBSERVATIONAL APPROACHES

In addition to the managers' ratings of quality of life through POET, Real Life Options wanted to gather more in-depth information on a sample of residents in relation to the support provided to them and the quality of life to which this support contributed. They therefore worked with the Health Services Management Centre at the University of Birmingham in completing the Adult Social Care Outcomes Tool (ASCOT) with one resident in each of the homes participating within the TORCH programme. This methodology has been developed over many years by the Personal Social Services Research Unit, is being promoted by the major social care research funding body in England (NIHR School for Social Care Research) and is the basis of the annual Adult Social Care Survey.[3]

ASCOT is based around established concepts regarding quality of life, which it separates into eight domains. The first four domains are the 'basic aspects of quality of life (personal cleanliness and comfort, accommodation cleanliness and comfort, food and drink, and feeling safe) and the next three domains are 'higher order' (social participation, occupation and control). The final domain (dignity) relates to the impact on people's self-esteem of the way the care and support are provided. ASCOT considers the quality of life of the person with support from social care services and also what their life would be like without social care support. This provides an idea of the type of benefits that they receive from receiving social care services. There are a variety of toolkits connected with ASCOT that have been adapted to reflect people's different living situations, life stages and abilities, and assessments against each domain can be gathered through the relevant combination of self-completion questionnaires, interviews and/or observations. An example of the type of analysis provided through the tool is given in Figure 12.2.

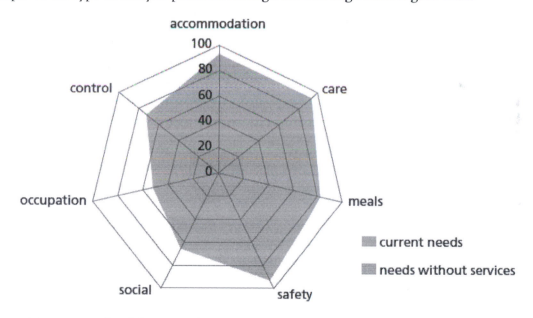

Figure 12.2 An example of the type of analysis achieved via the Adult Social Care Outcomes Tool
Blue shading signifies the person's quality of life achieved with the support of a social care sercice. Orange shading signifies quality of life without a service.

As none of the people living within the care homes would be able to complete the ASCOT questionnaire by themselves, the data was gathered as follows:

- observation of the resident over a four-hour period (including a meal)

- interview with resident (if they are able to participate)

---

3   See www.pssru.ac.uk/ascot for more information regarding ASCOT, accessed 4 July 2014.

- interview with key worker

- interview with family member (if they have regular contact with the resident).

This process enables the quality of life of the resident to be assessed against the aspects outlined above and also provides rich data regarding the lives of residents and their interactions with staff (see the case study below). The University of Birmingham provided training to staff members of Real Life Options regarding ASCOT and supported them on applying the approach to the sample of residents. The ASCOT assessors undertook the ASCOT assessment on a home in which they were not working. This provided a baseline of the current quality of life of the individuals living in the homes and also the practice within the homes. The ASCOT process will be completed 12 months later to assess what differences, if any, have been achieved. The findings of the ASCOT assessments were also fed back to the managers and staff teams within the homes so that they could reflect on how they are working and identify potential areas for improvement.

Paula's story: Example of Adult Social Care Outcomes Tool observation summary with regard to the aspect 'Control over daily life'

Observation

There were no instances in which Paula seemed to want to undertake an activity but was denied the opportunity by staff. Staff also allowed Paula to move at her own pace, and provided gentle encouragement to move in the direction of the doorway and hallway when asking her to go for her dinner or to be changed. Though it took some time for Paula to move out of the room, staff did not try to force her along.

Staff tried to engage with Paula in relation to finding out, for instance, if she wanted to go to another room, have a drink or listen to the radio or a tape; however, it was not clear whether she understood the question and/or whether staff understood her response, and therefore the staff member made the decision as they thought was in her interest (e.g. to have regular drinks, to listen to music) or what they perceived she may have communicated (e.g. she did not positively say she wanted the tape changed, so it was assumed that she must like what is currently being played).

Staff interview

Paula has some control over daily living but cannot control many aspects for herself. She is able, however, to move freely about the property and can choose whether to take part in activities or not by leaving the room where an activity is taking place. The staff want to take Paula to the library to help her choose her own audiobooks and tapes. Staff suggested that Paula could make choices and subsequently receive alternative options. It was not apparent from observations, however, that Paula was able to express preferences or understand alternatives.

Rating

Overall rating without services: High Needs
Overall rating with current services: Some Needs

Observational approaches

Bruce Lodge deployed two observational approaches to assess the impacts of their project. The first approach was through a Quality of Interactions (QUIS) methodology, which aims to capture the lived experience of people with dementia living or spending time in a care setting. QUIS captures the percentage of interactions that the resident undertakes under each of the following:[4]

- positive social and/or emotional interaction with staff, family, visitors or other individuals accessing the service

- positive personal care that attends to the individual's physical and personal care needs

- neutral care in which the main experience for the person is that of lethargy and boredom

- negative protective interactions in which staff members decide what is best for the individual and restrict or control what people can and cannot do in their private and communal areas

- negative restrictive interactions in which the restrictions placed on the individuals borders on (or is actually) abuse and is part of the overall culture of the service.

QUIS observations were undertaken in Bruce Lodge in March 2012 and again in July 2013 (Table 12.2). These data indicate that there had been marked increases in positive social and positive care interactions, and a reduction in neutral care and negative protective interactions. The increased scorings were based on observed interactions where there was a clear presence of genuine warmth being offered to individuals and lots of caring conversations. Staff laughed and joked with people and there were lots of hugs between staff and people living in the home. People were involved in activities they clearly enjoyed; for example, two men were being supported to set up a game of dominoes and another man was engaged in conversation with a volunteer about a recent outing where he had been on a boat.

Table 12.2 *Observed quality of interactions in Bruce Lodge*

Period of observation	Aspect of care				
	Positive social (%)	Positive care (%)	Neutral (%)	Negative protective (%)	Negative restrictive (%)
March 2012	0	17	70	13	0
July 2013	17	37	40	7	0

The second observational approach undertaken at Bruce Lodge was Dementia Care Mapping (DCM). This tool also aims to capture the experience of care from the standpoint of the person living with dementia, and it has gained international recognition as a reliable evaluation tool.[5] DCM captures minute by minute what the person is doing and their relative well-being. This is measured through their observed level of mood and the quality of their engagement with staff. The latter criterion is crucial due to its impact on the person's well-being, and understanding how staff interact with individuals reveals the underlying culture within the home (i.e. 'how we

---

4   Sheard, D. (2008) *Enabling: Quality of Life – An Evaluation Tool*. London: Alzheimer's Society.
5   See www.bradford.ac.uk/health/career-areas/bradford-dementia-group/dementia-care-mapping, accessed 4 July 2014.

do things around here'). Mapping was carried out in April 2012 and again for comparison in September 2013 by an independent expert in DCM.

The observations suggested that there had been a significant shift away from neutral care. In July 2012, the majority of time (91%) was spent with participants showing no signs of positive or negative mood and being only briefly engaged. In September 2013, however, the majority of time (72%) was spent with people showing considerable signs of either positive mood or engagement. People did still spend time in a neutral state, but the overall percentage of time spent in that state had been reduced from 91 per cent, in July, to just 23 per cent in September 2013. Furthermore, in September 2013 people spent 4 per cent of the observed time showing very high levels of well-being. This appears to indicate that people are experiencing higher levels of well-being and are spending less time in a neutral or passive state.

In addition to providing numerical-based data, DCM is a means to capture the conversations and experiences that really make a difference to a person's day.

Working Together for Change: building on person-centred reviews

In Chapter 5 we described a person-centred review process which brings together the provider, the person and their family and friends to reflect on progress in achieving the changes for the individual concerned, that is, identifying the top two things that are working for the person, the top two things that are not working and the top two things they would like to do in the future.

Working Together for Change (WTFC) is an eight-stage process designed to take information from person-centred reviews and use it to inform strategic decisions, including progress with achieving the aims of a change initiative (Box 12.5). At Bruce Lodge the leadership team took the first 12 person-centred reviews completed during the ISF programme and used the WTFC process to see what those reviews were telling them about what was working and not working for people overall, and what people wanted to do in the future. This is a powerful way to hear directly from people and their family about their experiences of the change, and what is working and not working from their perspective. This involved the whole leadership team, including Stockport Council and Borough Care Ltd, and other guests who may have a role in taking the overall learning forward. This included the person at Stockport Council who was taking a lead on the implementation of direct payments in residential care.

Box 12.5 Results of the Working Together for Change process

This is what the process indicated was working for people:

1. I am having more conversations and people are listening to me.

2. I am choosing what I do.

3. I am supported by staff who know me well.

4. I am doing something that feels useful.

5. I am reconnecting with people in my community.

6. I am doing more things that I enjoy.

7. I choose who to support and who supports me.

8. I am going out and doing things I want to do.

This is what the process indicated was not working for people:

1. I am less able to do things.
2. I am in poor physical health and cannot get out.
3. I don't get out as often as I want.
4. I don't always have enough money to do what I want.
5. I have important things that get lost.
6. I feel isolated when I'm having bed rest.
7. Sometimes I don't know what's happening.
8. I have no friends outside the home.
9. I miss being part of church life.

Here are the statements about what people wanted in the future:

1. I want to have a dog.
2. I want to get outside as much as possible.
3. I want to know what's happening next.
4. I want to have more company. I want to stay active and busy.
5. I want to stay well and on my feet.
6. I want to be involved in the church community more regularly.
7. I want Bruce Lodge to be my home until I die.

The group had clustered all the information from what was working, not working and important in the future, and then prioritised the themes to take forward into actions. These were the 'not working' aspects on which they decided to work:

- I feel isolated when I'm having bed rest.
- I have no friends outside the home.
- I don't get out as often as I'd like.
- I miss being part of my church community.
- I want to have a dog.

FROM CLUSTERS TO ROOT CAUSES AND SUCCESS, AND ACTION PLANNING

For each of these 'not working' themes we used a process called 'five whys' to identify the possible reasons for something not to be working. From our understanding about why this might be happening (possible root causes) and what we wanted to achieve (success from different perspectives), we could identify potential actions. We turned these into specific and measurable actions, with someone responsible, and used the same process for each of the prioritised five actions on which we wanted to work. This became the action plan for the next phase of our work together.

The leadership team found this is the clearest and the best way that individuals who are living with dementia and using the services at Bruce Lodge could inform us about how the service had developed and could further improve in the future. It also enabled them to contribute to the business planning for the whole of Borough Care Ltd. WTFC means that strategic plans can be created and reviewed without using focus groups, and without using questionnaires, but rather by taking the information directly from what people supported by Borough Care Ltd are saying about their lives in their person-centred reviews. Going forward, the manager plans to use WTFC annually to develop the service, and there is also an opportunity to carry out this process not just for a single care home (in this case Bruce Lodge) but also to aggregate the information from all of the care homes across Borough Care Ltd and use it to inform strategic business planning on an annual basis.

Conclusion

This chapter has highlighted that different methods and tools can be used to determine whether ISFs have led to the improvements in practice and quality of life that have been sought. They also enable organisations to discover how the change process has been experienced by different stakeholders and identify ways to make this process better.

We have now learned about how ISFs can be used as part of a person-centred process which enables individuals to be more in charge of their life and thereby achieve their personal goals, and the organisational changes that are necessary to implement ISFs successfully. In Chapter 13 we look to the future of health and social care services and the role that ISFs could play in these new opportunities and challenges.

ISFs: Moving to the Future

Chapter 13

ISFs: Beyond Block Contracts

Introduction

The starting point for many of the organisations were block contract arrangements in which a commissioner purchased a number of places within a residential care home or supported living scheme and then identified people who could be suitably supported in these settings. Most of these arrangements were linked to the closure of long-stay hospitals for people with a learning disability or mental health problem. With the closure of such facilities, there are likely to be less block contract arrangements in the future; however, this does not mean that there are not opportunities for ISFs to facilitate change. Bruce Lodge and the Look Ahead rehabilitation service are both examples of services which have been developed separately to a hospital closure programme but for which ISFs have proved to be a constructive tool.

Looking to the future, it is clear that there likely will be a number of key features of policy and the environment:

- Public-sector resources will be stretched due to rising demand related to improved medical care and overall life expectancy.

- Successful transition from children to adult services will be key to facilitate a greater independence and quality of life in adulthood.

- Public-sector funding will increasingly be paid through individual payment mechanisms in which the person receiving support, and their families or circle of support, have greater control and flexibility.

- More people will be expected to fund a significant portion or all of their care needs, possibly with the support of insurance companies.

- Lower-level types of support, such as home care and assistive technology, will be used to prevent admission to more expensive and intrusive options such as residential care and hospital treatment.

- More intensive types of support will seek to enable people to regain or develop independent living skills and their informal networks to reduce reliance on public-sector-funded services and improve quality of life.

In this chapter, we consider how the principles behind ISFs have been used to respond to these key issues through the experience of three additional organisations, in relation to self-funders (home care), transition and reablement.

ISFs and people who fund their own home care

Home-care packages can require multiple visits during the day and night, but there are many older people in particular who are supported to live in their own homes through a few hours per week. Often this home care complements support provided by their families, networks and community organisations such as places of worship and third-sector providers. Due to the current eligibility and charging processes (at least in England), many older people who receive such support pay for this care themselves. Therefore, an ISF is not necessarily required as the person holds their own care budget; however, as demonstrated by the organisations, being clear about the money is only one element of enabling people to have greater control over their care.

An example of how a provider used ISF principles to support someone with a relatively small care package can be found through the experiences of Hilda and United Response. (See the case study below for details of Hilda's situation when she became introduced to ISFs.) For United Response there were three key factors that encouraged the organisation to invest considerable thought and, therefore, resources in how they could better support someone who was purchasing a contract which cost less than £30 per week. First, they wanted to demonstrate what the most person-centred home care could look like, and for this to become 'simply the way we do business' whatever the size of the contract. Second, they wanted to build trust with Hilda. If they could provide her with staff that would be well matched to her, and support them to do an excellent job, then as Hilda needed more support, United Response might become her first choice to provide that support. Finally, if Hilda and her family were pleased with the service of United Response, they would be likely to mention it to other people, and this could lead to additional business.

Hilda's story:

Hilda was 92 years old, an avid film buff, who lived by herself near the coast. She was registered blind and in the early stages of dementia. Gill and Gill's daughters, Barbara and Rachel, supported her and stayed with Hilda a couple of nights per week. Hilda had great neighbours, too, Jean and Brian, who came to see her every day. Her daughter, Joan, lived in the United States. For Gill and Joan, and for Hilda too, there had been one-too-many near misses on the road to her local supermarket, and Hilda therefore needed help with her weekly shopping.

To understand what a person-centred home-care package would look like, United Response worked with Helen Sanderson Associates. A slimmed-down version of the person-centred planning process outlined in Section 2 was followed (Figure 13.1). This included a one-page profile for Hilda (specifying the outcomes and support she required for the service she was buying; Figure 13.2); a separate page with her specific outcome, her service specification and more detailed information on what good support looked like in relation to achieving her outcome (Figure 13.3); a matching template; and a one-page profile for the support worker.

The home-care package worked well for Hilda in a number of ways. She reported an increase in her overall well-being as she had the security of knowing that she could get out every week. She felt comfortable with her support worker and they often had a coffee together, which was a real highlight for Hilda. She also arranged specific things herself around what her and her support worker do together: for example, they went to the pharmacy for Hilda's medication check on one visit, which gave Hilda peace of mind. Her positive experience led to a number of word-of-mouth referrals through her and her network's contacts. Key to these improvements was the flexibility of her support worker, who was willing to change the days that she worked to respond to Hilda's preferences and to be a direct point of contact for the family. The support worker also tried to fit in with Hilda's existing home processes, for example, capturing reminders on her calendar in big writing. One issue that did arise was that Hilda became anxious about another support worker being introduced and preferred to cancel the call if her regular support was not available.

Sadly Hilda has since died; however, it was important that she was given the opportunity to have more control over her support over this period, and indeed even more as they were the final few months of her life. Despite the considerable work that this pilot involved for United Response, the organisation views this as being time and energy well spent.

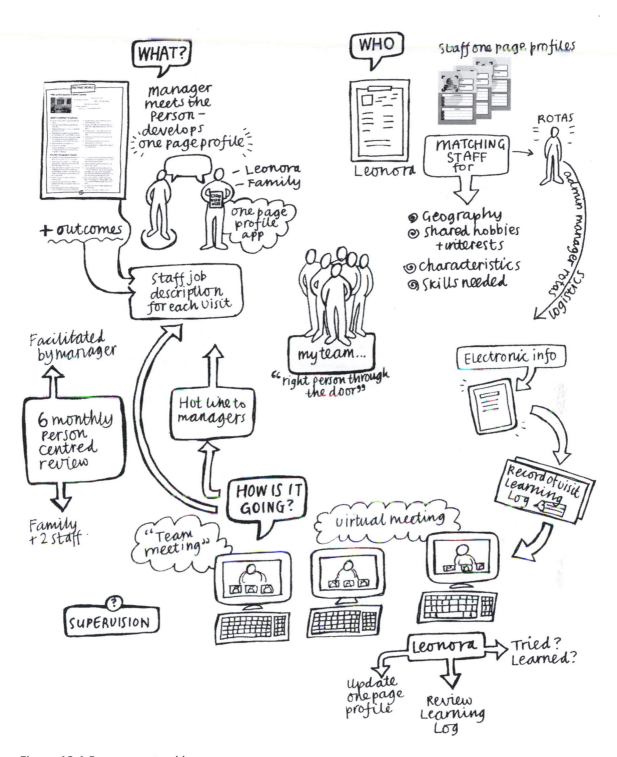

Figure 13.1 Person-centred home-care process

Hilda

What is important to Hilda

- Her family –Speaking to her daughter Joan and the family in the states twice weekly. Travelling
- to Pittsburgh to see Joan and Graham, and her grandchildren and great grandchildren when
- she can. Seeing Barbara her great niece every week, and Rachel a couple of times a month, and seeing Gill her niece.
- Chatting to her neighbours Jean and Brian everyday
- To go shopping every Sunday with Gill to Clevelys, have lunch in the café, and buys a new film on DVD
- Watching old films, and her favourite actors are William Holden, John Wayne and Audrey Hepburn.
- Watching soaps, in particular her favourite, Emmerdale, and then Strictly Come Dancing. She enjoys get the answers right when she watched Eggheads
- Her garden – it has raised beds, and Hilda makes new hanging baskets each spring
- Baking cakes and scones
- Going to Church, St James Layton, every week with Jean and Brian
- Listening to music on her CDs in the afternoon
- Her hairdresser who comes to the house each week to set her hair
- Reading the Sun each morning and then pushing it through Jean and Brian's letterbox by 11am for them to read
- Seeing her friend Muriel and ringing her when she cannot get round to see her
- For Barbara to do her 'office work'

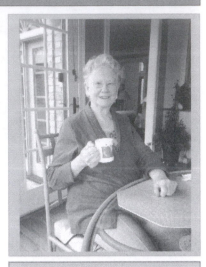

What we appreciate about Hilda

Great sense of humour,

Always upbeat,

Inspirational,

Incredibly organised,

Straight talking

How to support Hilda

- NEVER ask to borrow her DVDs or videos
- If you are visiting make sure you give her more than a weeks notice – she likes to prepare
- Hilda uses her magnifier and reader lamp when reading, always leave her magnifier on the coffee table by her chair
- Hilda manages the stairs well at home and will be irritated if you keep asking her if she is OK
- Never move furniture around as she will trip over it
- Never move her speaking clocks, she has one by her bed and one by the table by her chair
- Hilda is sensitive and will worry if she thinks she has offended you, avoid any jokes that may make her think she has upset you

Figure 13.2 Hilda's one-page profile

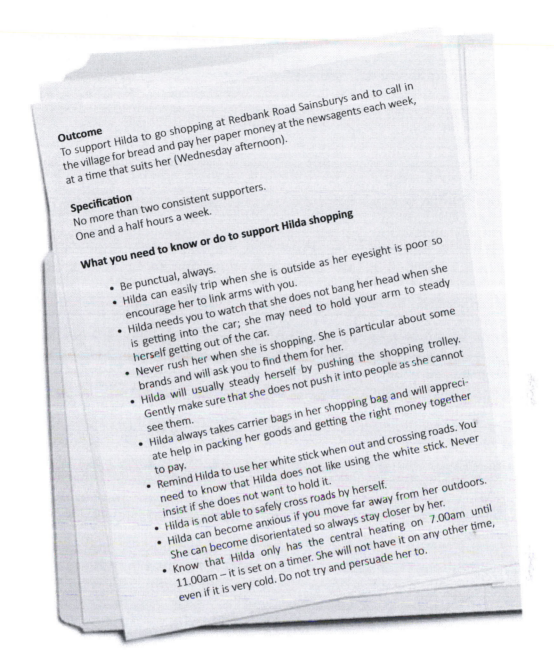

Outcome
To support Hilda to go shopping at Redbank Road Sainsburys and to call in the village for bread and pay her paper money at the newsagents each week, at a time that suits her (Wednesday afternoon).

Specification
No more than two consistent supporters.
One and a half hours a week.

What you need to know or do to support Hilda shopping

- Be punctual, always.
- Hilda can easily trip when she is outside as her eyesight is poor so encourage her to link arms with you.
- Hilda needs you to watch that she does not bang her head when she is getting into the car; she may need to hold your arm to steady herself getting out of the car.
- Never rush her when she is shopping. She is particular about some brands and will ask you to find them for her.
- Hilda will usually steady herself by pushing the shopping trolley. Gently make sure that she does not push it into people as she cannot see them.
- Hilda always takes carrier bags in her shopping bag and will appreciate help in packing her goods and getting the right money together to pay.
- Remind Hilda to use her white stick when out and crossing roads. You need to know that Hilda does not like using the white stick. Never insist if she does not want to hold it.
- Hilda is not able to safely cross roads by herself.
- Hilda can become anxious if you move far away from her outdoors. She can become disorientated so always stay closer by her.
- Know that Hilda only has the central heating on 7.00am until 11.00am – it is set on a timer. She will not have it on any other time, even if it is very cold. Do not try and persuade her to.

Figure 13.3 Hilda's service specification

ISFs and transition

Where transition works well, and education, health and care plans have a positive impact, it is likely that more young people will be able to use personal budgets to choose a different future. Jennie was supported by her mother, Suzie, and a circle of support, to use an ISF to support her transition from school to having paid work, a mortgage, exhibiting her art, and having her own support team.

Jennie's story:

Jennie is an active young person who participates in many sports and outdoor pursuits including walking, cycling and Zumba (a mix of dance and aerobics). She enjoys using her computer tablet to watch videos, listen to music and try out new applications, and is also interested in theatre, ballet and cinema. She has a great relationship with her mother, father and brother. She attended a specialist school for children with autism until she was 16 years old and then moved to a post-16 provision attached to her school until she was 19 years old.

When Jennie was at school, Stockport Council commissioned training for families in person-centred planning. Jennie's mother, Suzie, attended one of these courses and began to use person-centred planning with Jennie.

The prospect of leaving school and the staff with whom Jennie and her family had built up trusting relationships was a great concern to Suzie. Jennie was able to have regular short breaks from her family on a regular basis through children's services, and there was no guarantee that adult services would allow these breaks to continue. Beyond this support, Jennie and her family were also aware that leaving school and entering adulthood was an important transition for Jennie's whole life. Jennie had annual person-centred reviews at school, and one of the actions from her review in year 10 was to explore a circle of support to help Jennie and her family with transition.

Jennie's circle was made up of her family and friends. Jennie and the circle completed a Planning Alternative Tomorrows with Hope (PATH) person-centred plan at one of the early meetings. (This is a person-centred plan that specifically looks at the future and how the person can move towards their 'north star' dreams.) In planning for the future, it was also important to consider Jennie's parents and the role that they would be expected to play. These discussions led to the decision that Jennie would be supported to move into her own tenancy with a personal budget to purchase the care that she would require. Her parents were worried about the additional responsibility for them if they managed the budget on her behalf, particularly if this required employing and overseeing the work of care staff. The circle therefore opted for an ISF, in which the provider of the support would hold Jennie's personal budget.

Stockport Council had developed a Resource Allocation System (see Chapter 2) to calculate the budget that would be available for adults with eligible social care needs. To agree to allocate this money to Jennie, the Stockport Council required a support plan which would confirm what outcomes were important to her and how the personal budget would be used to achieve these outcomes. Jennie's Essential Lifestyle Plan and PATH contained most of the background information required to guide the development of her support plan. Key to this was for Jennie to have her own accommodation, and a housing specification was drawn up to identify what the essential features of her new accommodation should be (see Box 13.1).

Box 13.1: Jennie's housing specification

Essential:

- To live on her own with support staff and to have a bedroom for staff to sleepover in.

- To live close to her family in Stockport – within a ten-mile radius of their house.

- To live in a safe community, and for the house to have good security.

- To part own her home – and have this security (rather than being a tenant).

- To have a light, airy environment to meet Jennie's sensory needs.

Desirable:

- A garden.

- A room to have time away from support staff where she can do her art.

- Close to local amenities – cinema, swimming pool, train station, library etc.

Her circle of support helped develop her 'perfect week', which included a community map of the places that were important for her to visit and her relationship circle. This informed Jennie's support plan. The initial plan was more expensive than her personal budget would allow, and therefore the Just Enough Support process (see Chapter 4) was used to think through which other community resources and personal networks could be drawn upon. This included Jennie staying with her mother or father every weekend, which meant that her budget only had to pay for five days support and carefully assessing her support needs at night. This led to agreement that she would initially have additional funding to pay for a waking-night staff, but this would be reduced to a sleep-in night staff after three months. A decision-making agreement was part of her support plan, describing how Jennie would be involved in making choices over different aspects of her life.

Having agreed what was required, it was now time to put the housing and support plan into action. With the guidance of a housing advisor from a local provider called Independent Options, Jennie applied for a mortgage to purchase her own property. As she did not have the mental capacity to understand and therefore consent to a mortgage agreement, her mother had to apply to the Court of Protection so that she could become her legal deputy. This process took considerable effort and time, with considerable information being required at each stage. It was agreed, though, and a mortgage was set up to be funded through Jennie's benefits. An ideal flat had been found through a local housing association, and this flat was bought when the mortgage was agreed.

The additional responsibility – and therefore power – that managing the ISF would give meant that the right choice of provider was vital. Four potential providers were identified through Jennie's circle of support, and they all expressed an interest in holding the ISF on her behalf. The circle discussed the questions they would like to ask each provider. These questions were based around how they would work with Jennie, interact with her circle, engage Jennie and the circle in staff recruitment, and more general information about them as an organisation. The provider that was selected impressed the circle through their responses.

The circle wanted to be involved in the recruitment of staff to work with Jennie. The person-centred thinking tool 'matching staff' was used to help the circle consider the main characteristics of suitable staff, including their skills, interests and personality. A job description was drawn up from Jennie's Essential Lifestyle Plan which clarified what would be required of staff in relation to supporting Jennie, working with the family and circle, and employment with the provider. A bespoke advert was drawn up, with Jennie's mother and the manager from the organisation shortlisting potential candidates. There was then a three-stage interview process:

1. A group interview with the circle and the provider in which the candidates were introduced to Jennie and the organisation, and the candidates were asked to undertake individual and group tasks

2. A panel interview with each candidate

3. An informal interview in which Jennie met the candidates and they jointly participated in art activities.

Once staff were recruited, Jennie's mother led the training for the team on how best to support Jennie. This included spending time with Jennie to get to know her and her communication preferences and discussing her one-page profile and Essential Lifestyle Plan. Money from her personal budget was also used to pay for autism-specific training. Once Jennie moved into her flat, she had six monthly person-centred reviews with her family, her circle and the provider to ensure that there was a comprehensive review in which everyone's views were heard. She also had another PATH to look at her future now that she was living in her own flat, with her own support staff.

Now Jennie is paid to walk a dog each week, exhibits her art at a local art show and has a full week, supported by her staff team. Suzie, Jennie's mother, states:

> If you had said to me ten years ago that Jennie would be living independently in her own home, I would never have believed it. I was worried that she might be in an institutional setting or in supported living with people she didn't like or, worse still, didn't choose to live with. But now all the worry has gone, which has been amazing for me. Using Jennie's personal budget with a provider, through an ISF, has made all the difference.

ISFs and reablement

Since the late 2000's reablement services have been increasingly seen by local authorities and national government as a means to enable people to regain their independence following a health or social crisis. Reablement services were initially largely focused on working with a specific group of older people such as those who had been admitted to hospital, but in many areas they are now incorporated into the generic processes through which someone can access publicly funded social care services. There are many models of reablement services, with a common feature being that they support people intensively for 6–12 weeks in their own home. The way that reablement services provide support can prepare someone who needs to access services longer term to have an ISF in place, and in the short term, a more creative use of the public-sector resources could potentially facilitate better outcomes.

One organisation that has been trialling a more person-centred approach to reablement is Imagine, Act and Succeed (IAS). This organisation has been working in Northwest England for over 25 years providing community-based support to adults with a learning disability and their families. Following discussions with the organisation's local commissioner, IAS developed a reablement pilot in which the organisation would be allocated a £30,000 block of funding that could be used flexibly to respond to the needs of the people accessing the service. IAS used the principles of the 'new reablement journey'[1] and developed eight key principles of person-centred working in reablement (Box 13.2).

Box 13.2 Eight key principles of person-centred working in reablement

The eight key principles of person-centred working in reablement are as follows:

1. Reablement is a journey rather than a service and is not limited to six or eight weeks.

2. Reablement can be appropriate for anyone needing social care support.

3. People should be able to self-direct their reablement, that is, to exercise choice in how they are supported to achieve short- and longer-term outcomes.

4. There should be one person-centred 'harvesting' of relevant information.

5. Support planning should include outcomes that strengthen natural support networks and community involvement.

6. Plans to achieve short-term goals should be person centred; people will be involved in decisions about their support and will own the planning process.

7. People should have information about the resources available and agree a time frame to achieve specific outcomes.

8. People have a seamless experience with minimal 'hand offs' between professionals or services.

The service has been able to apply the principles within a new reablement journey (Figure 13.4). This involves developing a one-page profile and undertaking a 'what's working and what's not working' session with the person and their family to identify the current issues. Crucially, this session is completed within 24 hours of the referral and captures information regarding the person's assets and strengths as well as their support needs. This can lead to people deciding that they do not actually need any external support; those that do are matched to a suitable reablement worker. Progress is reviewed weekly, with a formal meeting held after three weeks with the care manager or referrer present. If someone requires longer-term support at the point of discharge, the person-centred information regarding the individuals is used to develop a support plan funded through a personal budget. This could be held by a provider in the form of an ISF, by the local authority or by the person as a direct payment. The reablement team also keeps in contact with people who do not receive further services to ensure that their situation has not deteriorated and that they are able to maintain that level of independence.

---

1   Pitts. J., Sanderson, H., Webster, A. and Skelhorn, L. (2011) *A New Reablement Journey*. Available at www.helensanderson associates.co.uk/media/52336/reablementfinalreport.pdf, accessed on 12 June 2014.

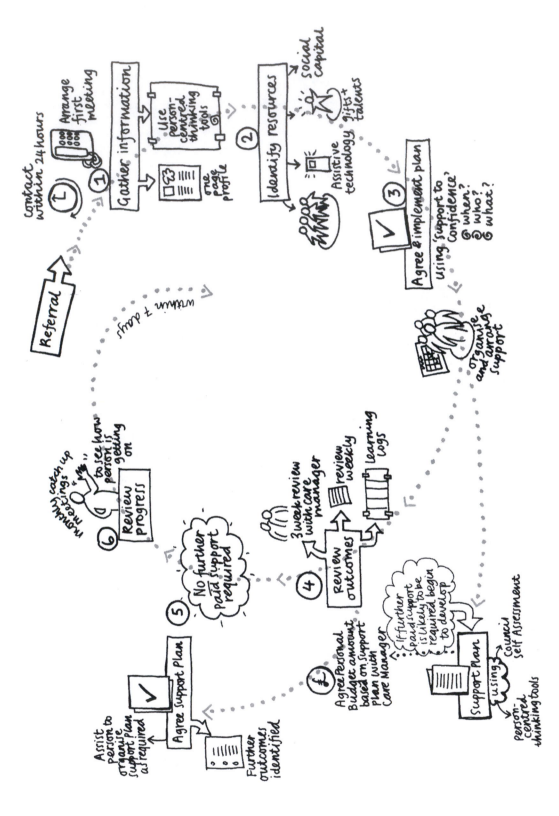

Figure 13.4 The new reablement journey. (From Pitts and Sanderson)[2]

2   Pitts *et al.* (2011).

The pilot project has been able to build upon the previous commitment and experience of IAS in delivering more person-centred services. Just Enough Support has been of particular relevance through ensuring that people are provided the support they need whilst not undermining their personal resilience and networks. Also key has been a trusting relationship with the commissioner and care management team. Despite the considerable experience of IAS, the organisation has found that the move to reablement has required it to work at a different pace which, in turn, requires support workers to believe in focusing on outcomes and enabling people to draw upon their own resources.

Rebecca's story

Rebecca is 18 years old and lives with her family. She has recently left college and wanted to develop the confidence to do more for herself, making links with her community and having friendships and a wider social network. She was referred to the reablement team by her care manager to provide support to develop that independence and for her to feel more connected within her community.

The reablement team leader, Dawn, met with Rebecca and her family to plan how this could be achieved. Dawn needed to establish what was working and what was not working, and she needed to make some changes and to agree some actions on how to implement them. Dawn identified well-matched staff who would support Rebecca during the coming weeks.

The team worked with Rebecca and her mother on a daily basis initially to support Rebecca to do more for herself – things she could do and things she could learn with support, advice and encouragement, when needed. When they were satisfied that Rebecca was confident in what she could do and her self-esteem had grown, the next step was to look at what was going on within her local community in which she could get involved. Rebecca started a cookery class to further develop her independent living skills and soon had something she was involved in most days of the week that enabled her to meet people and have fun. Initially Rebecca had support at each event to ensure she felt confident and comfortable. Her reablement team then worked with her on travel with the aim of her using the bus independently. Her support staff took steps back when appropriate as her skills and confidence grew. This gradual reduction in support followed weekly reviews which took place to check how things were going from everyone's perspective and to check that Rebecca felt ready for the next step.

The outcome was that Rebecca no longer needed support by staff either for travelling or attending the community-based events, something she achieved within a shorter timescale than originally anticipated. Rebecca's reablement journey ran for four weeks with a planned phased reduction over the final two weeks. Now with only a few hours of personal-assistant support when needed, for shopping and getting to places that are difficult by bus, Rebecca's reablement support has enabled her to develop into a confident young woman with the skills that are needed for her future, along with an active social life with opportunities to meet lots of people and the ability to maintain those friendships and develop new ones.

Conclusion

The future of ISFs will go beyond deconstructing block contracts and offering greater choice in congregate settings. It is likely that more people with personal budgets will make the same choice as Suzie and Jennie, that is, use their budget to purchase support from a provider. ISFs will also benefit, and be attractive to, people who fund their own services and support, young people who are eligible for funding as they leave school and people who need support leaving hospital. Although these ISFs may be called different names in the future, the principles of greater choice and control by knowing what funding one is entitled to, and deciding how to spend it, should remain intact.

Chapter 14
Overall Learning

Introduction

The organisations that have contributed their experiences to this book have all been committed to implementing the principles of personalisation for many years. Despite their best efforts, they recognised that to achieve these principles in practice and truly provide person-centred support, they still needed to do more, and that this would require further radical change. Through their experiences we have learned that ISFs can be used to generate this positive change for people who rely on health and social care services to sustain their health and well-being. This change is achieved through the implementation of ISFs being a process which enables staff and their organisations to put individuals at the heart of everything they do – in the minute-to-minute interactions between staff members and the individuals that they support, in the day-to-day management of services, such as the coordinating of rotas, prioritisation of resources, recruitment and training of staff and in the overall culture and accountability of the organisations.

ISFs have been used by these organisations to improve support within a wide range of services, including residential care, supported housing and domiciliary care. ISFs have begun to transform the lives of older people, those with mental health problems and people with a learning disability, and to be relevant for young people leaving school and those who are at the end of their life. Successfully implementing ISFs is not an easy task, though, and it requires sustained commitment from across the organisation over many months, if not years; however with good coordination, inspirational leadership and a willingness to engage with staff and other stakeholders, it is possible for the changes to succeed.

What have we learned?

We asked each of the organisations to reflect on their lessons learned, and to suggest ten key messages that they would share with other organisations that are interested in developing ISFs at scale and in all sorts of services. The information they provided was synthesised into the following 12 key lessons regarding ISFs:

START WITH WHAT SUCCESS LOOKS LIKE AND HOW YOU WILL KNOW IF YOU ACHIEVE IT

Establish your criteria for success at the outset, based on what you want to achieve for the people you support and for your organisation. One approach to this used by half of the organisations was to develop a one-page strategy to concisely communicate what success looks like from the perspectives of people supported, the workforce and the organisation overall.

HAVE A LEADERSHIP TEAM AND SUFFICIENT PROJECT MANAGEMENT

Certitude stressed the importance of a tight project management process (including an identified project manager) to ensure changes are achieved. They also suggested that having a leadership team that involved key people, for example, the finance team, not only helps to achieve the introduction of ISFs but also enables the leadership team to understand better the work of the organisation and the care staff to understand the finance role. This approach was used in most of the organisations, and including first-line managers was important.

Introducing ISFs on this scale is a major change that requires dedicated project management resources. It was more challenging when this was added to an operations manager's existing responsibilities.

Look Ahead stressed the importance of how the project plan needs to reflect robust risk management as well as accountability process.

DECIDE ON YOUR ALLOCATION SYSTEM EARLY AND MAXIMISE THE FUNDING AVAILABLE TO INDIVIDUALS

A key message from Dimensions was to develop your own views about how you would allocate a budget, what should constitute core services and what people can have under their personal control. Agree the ISFs before tackling any other issues, and explore if new technologies can be used to free up money that would otherwise be tied up in core costs.

EXCELLENT COMMUNICATION IS NECESSARY FOR EVERYONE

The organisations emphasised that ISFs are not about introducing a new procedure, and they require a shift in mindset and a more flexible approach. As United Response suggested, ISF and the ideas behind it need to be sold both inside and outside of provider organisations. United Response also reminds us that it requires providers to take a strategic view in that, whilst the ISF may not generate as much income as other, more traditional kinds of support work, it is part of the future and can allow organisations to develop a more diverse customer base.

There is still a lack of understanding about ISFs and their purpose and potential amongst people who use services, family members, social workers and providers; therefore, it is vital to provide people with clear information about the principles of personalisation, personal budgets and ISFs at the outset. Make sure that this extends to your partners; for example, Choice Support found that health and social work professionals do not always understand what ISFs entail, but getting them on board improves the person-centred planning process and helps to avoid potential resistance to individual budgets being agreed. Securing commitment from the local authority and having them publicly endorse the programme helps to reassure others that the changes are necessary and worthwhile.

The communication includes investing in partnerships, and United Response reminds us that a lack of trust between the commissioners and providers can delay or prevent progress towards more individualised funding. Dimensions, Bruce Lodge and Real Life Options invested in a range of creative ways to get the message across, with 'pub' quizzes and card games to help people check their understanding.

BE CLEAR ABOUT THE IMPLICATIONS FOR THE WORKFORCE

Build in sufficient time to adequately prepare, engage and inspire staff. People choosing their own staff is central to ISFs, and Dimensions encourages organisations to develop their organisational response to dealing with a member of staff whom nobody wants to support them. Help your staff understand that they must have their own personal offer for the people they are supporting. If they do not have one, help them to develop one.

DEVELOP AN APPROACH TO ROTA PLANNING THAT PUTS THE PEOPLE YOU ARE SUPPORTING AT THE CENTRE

One of the ways you can tell whether any organisation is really delivering choice and control around what people do and who supports them is to look at the rotas. Dimensions invested in its own time management system to make sure that rotas could be truly personalised. The majority of the organisations used the person-centred thinking tool 'matching support' to match the right staff member for each activity, and it is important to make sure this happens consistently.

INVEST IN COMPETENCE IN PERSON-CENTRED PRACTICES

This was a very strong theme – that the manager and the team should be familiar with person-centred thinking tools and should work towards becoming 'fluent' in them. Managers can use Progress for Providers to self-assess their level of competence and what support they need to improve, and this was used by almost all of the organisations.

SUPPORT YOUR MANAGERS – PROVIDE MORE THAN JUST TRAINING

Choice Support made the important point that formal training needs to be followed up with practice-based support which helps staff members to apply the theory into their work. Bruce Lodge supported staff and managers mainly through on-site coaching, and Real Life Options invested in a significant training and support programme for managers. The clear message is that just sending staff on training is not enough to create the competence and changes in practice that ISFs require from managers.

EMBED SUPPORT PLANNING WITHIN YOUR EXISTING PAPERWORK AND SYSTEMS

Integrate the person-centred information required for support planning within your personal files for individuals, rather than it being seen as a separate initiative. Look Ahead reflected on how important it was to build the individual allocation planned and actual spend into Care Programme Approach reviews, and meetings with care coordinators and team meetings. Certitude and Dimensions in particular stressed the importance of integrating person-centred practices within the information recorded about individuals, and the dangers of ending up with two sets of information – one for ISFs and the existing information.

HAVE WAYS TO DISCOVER WHAT IS WORKING AND NOT WORKING ABOUT THE CHANGE, FROM DIFFERENT PERSPECTIVES

Getting feedback about how the change is happening, and what is working and not working from different perspectives, is vital to keep adjusting the project plan to reflect what you are learning. Having intentional processes for getting feedback from people, families, staff, managers, professionals and the project team was emphasised in particular by Real Life Options and Bruce Lodge. Dimensions recommends that organisations approach challenges openly and resist the temptation to attribute blame and fault. You will learn much more and achieve positive change more quickly by clarifying your expectations and engaging in honest and open dialogue.

BE REALISTIC AND CELEBRATE SUCCESSES AND EARLY WINS

As well as hearing what is not working and what you need to change, it is important to create, celebrate and share early wins, and invest in stories and examples being written up and shared. Be realistic about your progress and achievements. Major change to working practices takes courage, determination and time.

TRACK AND EVALUATE YOUR PROGRESS

Choice Support and Real Life Options suggest that it is helpful to have an external body, such as a university, to evaluate the process and impact, as they bring evidence and objectivity about what has been achieved. Bruce Lodge did before-and-after evaluations, and many organisations used Progress for Providers to help keep the changes on track.

Index

A Practical Guide to Delivering Personalisation

Person-Centred Practice in Health and Social Care

HELEN SANDERSON AND JAIMEE LEWIS

Paperback: £21.99 / $35.00
ISBN: 978 1 84905 194 1
240pp

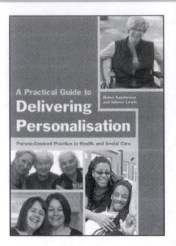

Personalisation means people, their families and carers having choice and control over their support on a day-to-day basis. To deliver personalised services, professionals and carers need to do more than just hand over financial control: they need to know what is important to a person, the best way to support them, how they communicate and how they make decisions.

This book will show how to deliver personalisation through simple, effective and evidence-based person-centred practice that changes people's lives and helps them achieve the outcomes they want. It covers why person-centred practice is relevant to the personalisation agenda and what person-centred thinking and person-centred reviews are, introducing the tools that can help you carry them out. It also explores the relationship between person-centred plans and support plans, and how person-centred practice can be used in the journey of support through adulthood – from prevention or the management of long-term health conditions to reablement, recovery, support in old age and at the end of life. There is also a chapter on taking a person-centred approach to risk.

This is an essential guide for all staff in health and social care including service providers, managers, practitioners and students.

Helen Sanderson is CEO of Helen Sanderson Associates and Director Emeritus of the International Community for Person-Centred Practices. She has been closely involved in the development of person-centred thinking and planning in the UK over the last 15 years, and has written extensively on person-centred thinking, planning, community building and Individual Service Funds. HSA were runners up with Borough Care in the National Dementia Awards 2012 in the innovation category. **Jaimee Lewis** is strategic communications adviser to the Think Local, Act Personal Partnership, the sector-wide commitment to transforming adult social care that follows on from Putting People First. She has worked on communicating the personalisation agenda for several years, following her appointment as an advisor to the Department of Health's individual budgets pilot programme in 2006.

Creating Person-Centred Organisations

Strategies and Tools for Managing Change in Health, Social Care and the Voluntary Sector

STEPHEN STIRK AND HELEN SANDERSON

Paperback: £29.99 / $49.95
ISBN: 978 1 84905 260 3
336pp

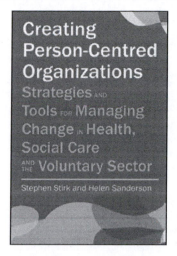

Person-centred thinking and planning are approaches that enable people using social care and health services to plan their future, and use a personal budget to commission personalised services.

Creating Person-Centred Organisations is a guide for organisations who want to deliver personalised services. Key issues covered include attending to the vision, strategy and business planning of the organisation, as well as organisational processes, culture and managing change. Drawing on the pioneering work of the social care charity United Response, the authors provide a wealth of practical tools and techniques to enable organisations within health, social care and the voluntary sector to use person-centred thinking tools and approaches to move towards becoming person-centred organisations.

This is an essential guide for managers and leaders within private, statutory and voluntary organisations.

Contents: Acknowledgements. List of Figures. Part 1. 1. Person-centred Organisations. 2. Person-centred Practices and Conventional Organisation Development. Part 2. 3. Vision, Mission, Values and Strategy. 4. Organisation Design. 5. Working Together. 6. Creating a Person-centred Culture. 7. Leadership. 8. Human Resources. 9. Person-centred Team Working. 10. Enabling Risk. 11. Measuring and Improving Quality. 12. Managing Change. 13. Conclusion. Appendix 1. Progress for Providers. Appendix 2. Progress for Providers for Managers. Endnotes. About the Authors. Index.

Stephen Stirk is Director of Human Resources for the social care charity United Response. He has had over 30 years' experience in human resources, organisation development and line management positions, including specialism in organisation design and development with GlaxoSmithKline. **Helen Sanderson** is CEO of Helen Sanderson Associates and Director Emeritus of the International Community for Person-Centred Practices. She has been closely involved in the development of person-centred thinking and planning in the UK over the last 15 years, and has written extensively on person-centred thinking, planning, community building and Individual Service Funds. HSA were runners up with Borough Care in the National Dementia Awards 2012 in the innovation category.

Person-Centred Teams

A Practical Guide to Delivering Personalisation Through Effective Team-work

HELEN SANDERSON AND
MARY BETH LEPKOWSKY

Paperback: £19.99 / $32.95
ISBN: 978 1 84905 455 3
168pp

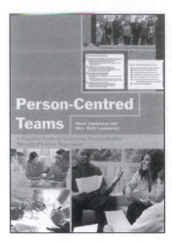

Person-Centred Teams provides much-needed guidance on person-centred working following the roll out of personalisation and personal budgets across health and social care.

In order to deliver personalisation you need to work with staff in person-centred ways. Straightforward and easy-to-read, this practical guide describes how to do this by developing a person-centred team using person-centred practices. The authors outline their model for developing a team, and how information is recorded in a person-centred team plan. They explain:

   Purpose - how to clarify a team's purpose

   People - what managers need to know about each team member, and how one-page profiles can help

   Performance - how to clarify service users' expectations of a team's services, and assess whether or not these are being met

   Process - how person-centred practices can aid teamwork and help your team deliver

   Progress - how to continuously improve teamwork and performance

Each section features clear illustrations and examples from teams to enable you to develop a person-centred team plan and work together in person-centred ways.

This guide is essential reading for service providers, managers, practitioners and students in the health and social care fields, as well as person-centred planning coordinators and user-led organisations.

Helen Sanderson is CEO of Helen Sanderson Associates and Director Emeritus of the International Community for Person-Centred Practices. She has been closely involved in the development of person-centred thinking and planning in the UK over the last 15 years, and has written extensively on person-centred thinking, planning, community building and Individual Service Funds. HSA were runners up with Borough Care in the National Dementia Awards 2012 in the innovation category. **Mary Beth Lepkowsky** has been building internal capacity of emerging leaders, front-line supervisors, middle managers and organization executives for more than 30 years. As Founder and Principal Consultant of Pathways Facilitation Services, Mary Beth provides leadership training, facilitation, continuous improvement and strategic planning support for non-profit and public sector organizations. She is also Assistant Director of Training and Organizational Development of Tri-Counties Regional Centre, a California non-profit that provides person and family centred supports and services for individuals with intellectual and developmental disabilities. She is a certified trainer of the international Learning Community for Person Centred Practices and a Certified Professional Coach. Mary Beth lives with her husband and two sons in Solvang, California.

Personalisation in Practice

Supporting Young People with Disabilities through the Transition to Adulthood

SUZIE FRANKLIN WITH HELEN SANDERSON
FOREWORD BY NICOLA GITSHAM

Paperback: £13.99 / $24.95
ISBN: 978 1 84905 443 0
128pp

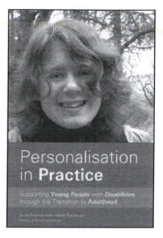

This book demonstrates very clearly how the personalisation of support and services works in practice. The authors describe how Jennie, a young person with autism and learning difficulties, was supported through the transition from school to living independently using simple, evidence-based person-centred planning tools. Jennie's story illustrates the importance of quality person-centred reviews, dispels the many myths surrounding Individual Service Funds and personal budgets and demonstrates how families, schools and other agencies can work collaboratively to help young people with disabilities move into adulthood with more choice and control over their lives, and with better life prospects. Practical pointers for readers to apply to their own circumstances are included, and the book contains helpful examples of the key person-centred thinking tools.

Anyone involved in supporting children and young people with disabilities as they approach adulthood, including parents and carers, SENCOs, teachers, social workers and service providers, will find this to be essential reading. More generally, it will be an informative resource for those seeking a better understanding of how personalisation and person-centred planning work in practice.

Suzie Franklin is the mother of Jennie, a young woman with autism and learning difficulties. She works in the voluntary sector, helping other families of children and young adults with autism to advocate for themselves and learn about their rights and entitlements. She has run training and parent workshops on a variety of topics related to autism, and is an advocate of person-centred planning. She runs training on person-centred thinking tools to help families, local authorities and other agencies provide better support and services for people with disabilities. **Helen Sanderson** is CEO of Helen Sanderson Associates and Director Emeritus of the International Community for Person-Centred Practices. She has been closely involved in the development of person-centred thinking and planning in the UK over the last 15 years, and has written extensively on person-centred thinking, planning, community building and Individual Service Funds. HSA were runners up with Borough Care in the National Dementia Awards 2012 in the innovation category.

CPSIA information can be obtained at www.ICGtesting.com
Printed in the USA
BVOC01s0517151014.

370581BV00009B/3/P